ACKNOWLEDGEMENTS

This book is dedicated to my wonderful sons Joseph and Jordan,"You are the light of my life and inspiration for all that I do. Thank you for believing in me and for being so patient whilst I was researching and writing this book. I love you always and forever."

To Terri, "your friendship changed my life, thank you for always being there for me."

My deepest gratitude to my assistant copy editor Susan Pereira for helping me complete this book in time for the deadline. "I am thrilled the diet improved your health and well being."

To my parents for the passing down their love of good healthy food. It is wonderful to know this diet has been beneficial to you both as an energy boosting tool.

"Gratitude is when memory is stored in the heart and not in the mind" Lionel Hampton

INDEX

INTRODUCTION

The Food Voice Diet is a spiritual, mental and body approach to weight reduction. Your food voice is the silent commentary operating in your head guiding food choices. If your food voice is tuned in and working well, you receive suggestions to consume healthy food in the right quantity. An imbalance, however, causes cravings and binges caused by faulty messages directing you to eat. This voice can run all day instead of at meal times becoming demanding and insistent. This book explains why using will power against foods you attempt to deny yourself is doomed to failure. If your food voice insists upon a particular food you will eventually give in. There are various reasons why your food voice is out of tune causing weight issues. Find out why you are getting messages to overeat the wrong food and learn how to instruct your food voice to help instead of sabotaging your weight loss efforts. The Food Voice Diet also improves energy levels, it is an effective energy boosting diet if weight loss is not an issue or you have reached your goal weight and wish to maintain your success.

Your habits, emotions and behaviour unlock the first key to acquiring a new healthy food voice, transforming your old habits which are urging you to consume the wrong type of foods. Once you learn which factors are controlling your food intake you will be empowered. Where does the urge to eat all the wrong foods come from? You may well assume that you are to blame, but it is actually far removed from what is going on behind the scenes. No diet will work if you have existing programming ruining your efforts despite a desire to lose weight. Diet books tend to underestimate the power food has over you by expecting you to lose weight without the correct tools. Ignoring this power is unfair, as you will believe you have failed and it is all your fault. After reading this book, you will be able to let go of any guilt as you will understand how you have been programmed and seduced by addictive food. Once you also learn how the other weight reduction blocks can be resolved, guilt will belong to the past along with your excess weight.

This diet will teach you the following key steps to discover your healthy, slimmer food voice.

Key 1
How to change your existing learnt behaviours and eating habits from childhood, culture and
environment, preventing you from successful permanent weight loss.

Key 2
How the brain can take control of our food choices. Knowledge is power, you will learn how to eat to ensure you remain in control. Addictive food can hijack your food voice keeping you enslaved to consume this food, whilst sapping your energy and causing weight gain.

Key 3
Which foods and eating habits cause fat storage instead of fat burning? Learn how to train your food voice to help you to burn excess fat.

Key 4

How to change limiting beliefs that keep you in the weight gain trap. This is the path to long-term weight loss. What food voice messages are running in the background working against you?

Key 5

The diet programme is based on low carbohydrate consumption in relation to your personal level of activity. Carbohydrate excess is stored and turned to fat. This extra fat can affect the liver and other bodily functions causing cravings, disrupts hunger and fullness signals resulting in overeating. Learn how to eat to lose weight, boost energy, restore health and mental balance.

This book is divided into two sections, the first half covers weight related **problems** in keys 1-5. The second part focuses on the **solutions.**

Being overweight affects so many areas in our lives such as self-esteem, relationships, parenting, careers and can erode all areas of our happiness, health and peace of mind. Having a food and weight issue is emotionally and physically draining, not to mention stressful. Weight gain tends to go hand in hand with lack of energy. The Food Voice Diet improves energy levels whilst you lose weight, setting you up to be fully able to enjoy the new lighter you. Slimmer but exhausted is not part of the philosophy of this book. If you have a food voice that is demanding sugar and carbohydrate and a constant supply of fattening food or you feel out of control with your eating this book is for you.

OBESITY AND STATISTICS

Feeling trapped by overeating and food issues, creates a
life of unhappiness as weight gain affects us negatively in
so many ways. Failed dieting has become an expectation as
more information via the media bombards us with stories of
obese people who are struggling to lose weight to save their
lives. Statistics reveal that obesity is increasing to epidemic
proportions worldwide as it claims victims from toddlers,
teens and upwards including the elderly. Statistics say by 2015
fifty percent of the world population will be obese. Countries
such as China, Mexico and India had previous problems
with malnutrition, but now surprisingly have serious obesity
problems.

The underlying message regarding a solution to obesity seems
to be one of hopelessness and failure, which indicates that
food actually has extensive power over us. It is a fact that
food can control us if we do not know how to prevent it. This
book will explain what you can do to take your control back
by knowing all the facts about how various food issues work
in order to avoid the pitfalls.

It does seem bizarre that certain foods can be the cause of so
many health related problems. Food looks so innocent and
harmless leading us to view food as a path to feeling good,
enjoyable tastes and experiences, enabling us to ignore all the
facts regarding the damage it is doing to our health. Food is
so appealing, however, what we see with our eyes bears no
relevance to the damage it can do to our waistline. Do not let
your eyes fool you as visually food resembles pure pleasure
but it has a very large punch when it gets to work on your

fat cells. What you need to know is what makes you choose the wrong food in the first place before any new eating programme will work for you properly.

There is a desperate need to be set free from the prison of food entrapment. I wanted to get to the bottom of this dilemma which is seriously affecting millions of people. I decided to find out why this is happening and what is really affecting our ability to control and prevent this problem from harming more and more people each year. Obesity, weight gain and food addictions are such complex issues because food consumption is essential for survival. Other addictive substances such as alcohol and drugs are avoidable, but if you have an eating problem, you have to deal with it permanently for the rest of your life.

KEY FACTS FROM THE WORLD HEALTH ORGANISATION (WHO) 2013

- Worldwide obesity has nearly doubled since 1980.

- In 2008, more than 1.4 billion adults, 20 and older, were overweight. Of these people, over 200 million men and nearly 300 million women were obese.

- 35% of adults aged 20 and over were overweight in 2008, and 11% were obese.

- 65% of the world's population live in countries where overweight and obesity kills more people than underweight.

- More than 40 million children under the age of five were overweight in 2011.

- **Obesity is preventable.**

THE NATIONAL HEALTH SERVICE (NHS) 2013

Being obese can lead to serious health problems, as well as shorten your life expectancy.
It is estimated that there are around 35, 000 obesity-related deaths in England each year. This accounts for one in every 16 deaths.

Being overweight or obese can increase your risk of health problems, including: high blood pressure (hypertension), this is a major risk factor for developing a serious cardiovascular disease (conditions that can affect the circulation of blood around the body).

- Infertility
- Type 2 diabetes
- Many types of cancer
- Heart disease, stroke
- Asthma
- Osteoarthritis – a condition that affects the joints
- Back pain
- Depression
- Liver and kidney disease
- Sleep apnoea – a condition that causes interrupted breathing during sleep

- Gastro-oesophageal reflux disease

If you are obese, you are also more likely to develop complications in pregnancy, such as gestational diabetes or pre-eclampsia (which is when a woman experiences a potentially dangerous rise in blood pressure during pregnancy)

I am sure many of these facts concerning the health risks of being overweight are not all together new to you. The trouble is that despite the negative implications of this data, many people remain compelled to eat the same problem foods causing these medical issues, due to habits and the lack of awareness of other factors such as the brain chemistry of addictive foods. It is disheartening and distressing if the diet advice you have received up to now has not worked for you.

What if you discovered:

1. You are being controlled by certain foods.

2. You have hidden programming which sabotages weight loss.

3. Your excessive hunger comes from a faulty brain message service.

4. You are storing fat because your fat cells cannot hear vital fat burning messages?

The Food Voice Diet is akin to resetting your brain computer system, giving you access to weight loss software. The new software will override the old programming which featured overeating, cravings, binges and the yearning for junk food. You will need to learn some new information, work out what needs to be reset, make some new food choices and remember how to keep the new programme working and in good order. This diet programme helps you not only to lose weight, but is your personal guide to keeping the weight off permanently. The Food Voice Diet will help to alleviate many of the above mentioned health issues listed by The World Health Organisation and National Health Service as many of the diseases mentioned can be prevented with weight loss and healthy eating.

I wanted solutions to the following issues:

- Why typical diets do not work in the long run despite the knowledge available from the internet, magazines and books? Why, with all this data so readily available worldwide, is it so difficult for people to lose weight?

- What is making us fat and keeping us that way? Why is lack of energy another major modern day problem?

- Why is obesity on the increase despite advances in medicine and science? Why are certain foods addictive? What causes binge eating? What drives an excessive appetite?

- What is relevant in your life with regard to your weight gain? What is not working for you? Do you have the knowledge about what to eat, but you find yourself eating the wrong foods over and over again?

- Why is temptation and thinking about certain foods such a big issue despite the negative effects it has on our lives when over weight?

- How to stop living in fear of food. Discover enjoyable nourishing foods you can eat without fear of piling on the pounds. Enjoy improved health and energy levels.

My mission is to provide a solution to give people peace from the fatness that literally seems to be attacking the human race like a huge virus. I want to eliminate this pain. I have spent the last two years researching medical and scientific data to find the cause for this effect. I can now introduce you to a way of eating and thinking which gives you peace from cravings and a constant annoying background food voice that will not shut up, encouraging you to eat weight gain foods. Glossing over the issue with diet plans and exercise does not help people get to the nitty-gritty of this problem. If calorie counting and low fat diets were solutions, they would be working, yet statistics prove the opposite.

If diet and exercise programmes are failing it is clear that the problem is much larger than we have been led to believe. Diets generally make weight loss seem so simple by suggesting we need to burn more calories by exercising, eat less and bingo, we lose weight. In theory it makes perfect sense, but in reality this is clearly not a successful remedy for the majority of sufferers. It is obvious that obesity and other weight related problems are more complicated and involve other issues that need to be addressed in order to find workable, long-term solutions. Weight management cannot be dealt with using the same old simplistic diet book advice, as decade after decade has not delivered successful results. Food has the power to be able to control not only our thoughts, but our actions, taste buds and our waistline. Food cravings and the use of certain foods to get through the day can take its toll as we pay a very high price for these indulgences. Fighting this powerful enemy needs a new approach and this book delivers solutions.

SIGNS YOUR FOOD VOICE IS OUT OF BALANCE

This book offers practical solutions for people who have a problem with overeating resulting from physical, emotional and other issues. If you are eating, focusing only on taste and the sensation of food, health is often the last thing on your mind in this state. Once we have eaten, food quickly disappears to the stomach. Food is out of sight and out of mind as far as the last meal or snack is concerned as though the rest of the body is none of our concern. We cannot see the damage certain foods are doing to our insides yet the results show on the outside such as weight gain, lack of energy, ill-health and skin problems. The following are signs that your food voice needs a tune up.

- Using food as a mood changer or distraction.
- Eating to punish yourself.
- To release tension and stress or to ward off feeling tired, having no energy.

- Difficult habit patterns such as eating whilst reading or watching television.
- Inability to stop eating when full.
- Food cravings for junk food.
- Thinking about food excessively. Obsessing. Only happy when eating
- Unable to stay on a healthy eating plan for more than a short space of time.
- Feeling out of control with eating behaviour.
- Overwhelming fear that you are unable to lose weight.
- To avoid dealing with problems or people
- Spending excessive time with food related pastimes.
- Withdrawal symptoms.
- Your tolerance to junk food has increased.
- You eat certain food brands to follow trends.
- Not eating the required nutrients your body needs.
- You spend more money on junk food than healthy food
- You have food related health issues such as obesity, metabolic syndrome, high blood pressure.
- You lack energy and feel lethargic.
- Excessive appetite

By making the changes suggested in this book, new food choices will benefit your whole body, not just your taste buds. The goal is to help you choose food that will not cause guilt, regret and negative feelings. You will be eating for nourishment and weight loss not to just feed cravings or emotions. Instead, you will experience waves of well being from eating healthier food, increased energy, weight reduction plus a sense of freedom and relief from an annoying and draining food voice. Knowing that the food you have just eaten is performing tasks on your behalf such as fat burning, repair, maintenance, circulation, heart health, brain function, building bones and good brain chemicals- connects food to your whole being. This is the correct pathway for you to become the master of your health and weight management.

If you have any of these issues, it is important to know that you are not weak willed, a glutton or a failure as you have previously learnt many of your poor food habits. I will explain step by step why you are having such a problem with food and weight gain and I will guide you to resolve this problem once and for all as this approach makes lasting change straightforward. Yes, you will have to make some effort to follow the steps and make the changes, but the solution is not as difficult as you may be thinking. If you have failed with weight loss before you may well be experiencing a lack of belief about a solution that will work for you. Take each step at a time and before you know it, you will have started on your journey of self-discovery as to what it takes to lose weight permanently.

THE AIMS OF THIS BOOK

- Learn how to change your food voice for lasting weight loss
- Informative yet easy to understand
- Limited science, physiology, anatomy facts and diagrams
- No case histories of people you do not know and whose weight loss success story bears no relevance to your life.

- Instructions and simple explanations as to why each step is important
- To motivate you to succeed
- Improve your health
- Lose stored fat not lean tissue.
- Improve energy levels

"That is what learning is. You suddenly understand something you've understood all your life, but in a new way" Doris Lessing.

No diet or eating programme will work for you in the long run unless you change the food beliefs, which are working against you. Every choice you make regarding the food you eat comes from such beliefs whether you are consciously aware or not. You may be working on a belief you learnt from childhood such as second helpings make you big and strong. If this belief no longer suits your waistline, your food voice needs to change this reminder at mealtimes. No one eats anything unless deep down there is a belief the food will make us happy in some way even if that happiness is very short lived and does not extend beyond the actual consumption of food. You may not be aware that you have these beliefs, but be assured they are there. I will help you to find these old beliefs and show you how to change them. I have created the 5 keys which have proven to be most successful for weight loss, controlling appetite, cravings and improving energy levels.

The Food Voice Diet gets to the actual cause of weight gain by providing you with a range of simple solutions that work from deep within you. All your power is inside you. To access it, all you have to do is follow the guidelines in this book to find the new food voice within. Food talks! Learn how to hear the sound of food which supports you. Imagine the day when you no longer hear the food you currently find so tempting beckoning you from your cupboards.

Having read all the causes of weight gain in keys 1-5 you can take the necessary steps to transform your body as you will possess the know how. There is no "one size fits all" diet plan and menu to suit everyone, but I have made every effort to consider the following needs and range of individuals that this book can truly help. Before starting this diet please seek the advice of your doctor if you have existing medical conditions or you are suffering from an eating disorder such as anorexia. However, I would add that booking a check up with your doctor is a good idea for anyone who is overweight as blood pressure and blood tests can detect any problems that need attention before you diet. This diet is suitable for:

- Men and women (excluding pregnant women, nursing mothers)
- Older teenagers (excluding those in high level sports)
- Normal weight but lacking energy
- Wanting to switch to a healthier diet
- For weight maintenance and post weight loss.
- Vegetarians (a wide variety of non animal protein sources must be included to ensure all the essential amino acids are consumed)
- People suffering from depression, type 2 diabetes, pre diabetes, ADHD, asthma, arthritis, fatty liver, fatigue,

high blood pressure, Alzheimer's disease, dementia, cardiovascular disease and other previously mentioned medical conditions.

Weight reduction in combination with limiting the consumption of sugar, junk food and trans fat can prevent and support numerous health and medical conditions. This diet is very flexible and easy to follow with special consideration to meals which fit into your social life, eating on the go, cooking for a family and preparing quick meals during a busy schedule. A diet should not add stress to your life, if it is taking too much time or causing you hassle then you will give up. Life is not a perfect picture postcard. There are some days when we are simply running against the clock, something upsetting or stressful crops up. During these times following a strict diet plan is the last thing on your mind. Not everyone enjoys cooking, this plan can support the basic and gourmet cook. Most of all this regime can help you make the necessary changes to your diet whilst living your life with its ups and downs. The diet can work around the speed at which you choose to apply to the diet changes. Certain people are fast responders and feel ready to go all out at full speed whilst others can only cope on cruise control for the first few weeks until they feel ready to make further adjustments. Having a certain goal such as a wedding or holiday gives you the necessary motivation to work quickly, however if this does not apply to you, do not worry just make the changes you can for now because once you start to lose weight and feel better the rest will come together for you. Taking time to adjust works well as long as the end goal of losing weight and eating healthier food does not fall by the wayside.

The new version of you awaits your discovery. Let us get inspired

THE FOOD VOICE DIET CAN HELP YOU

- Re-programme your food voice to help you lose weight.
- Reduce the desire to use food for emotional back up.
- Be in control of your food intake. Reduce the consumption of junk and processed food.
- Take your power back from food temptations.
- Eliminate quick fix dieting and change habits for life.
- Help you lose weight, but not feel constantly hungry.
- Change old beliefs about food issues and problems.
- Lose weight quickly.
- Lose weight permanently and rebalance your life.
- Eat to burn fat not add to fat storage
- Avoids lowering your metabolism making you less active and prone to weight gain.
- Reduce stress.
- Get rid of weight related guilt
- Eat nutrient rich foods
- Improve your energy levels.
- Improve mental health and well-being.

THE FOOD VOICE DIET IS NOT

- An over strict set of rules
- Fasting and calorie counting.
- A weighing portions diet
- Complicated

- Must follow a recipe plan
- A battle of will power
- Leaves you unsure how to eat once you have lost weight
- Reliant on buying low calorie brand meals
- Unrealistic and unsustainable
- Boring
- Just another diet book.

As a huge believer and follower of a low carbohydrate diet and after reading so many books and following this diet myself, I still found I had problems keeping to the diet for more than a few weeks. My extensive research enabled me to discover what the blocks were and why I was going off track. I was losing the weight and yet I was self-sabotaging why? Well, I was so focused on my weight goal that I placed food enjoyment low down on my list of priorities leaving me feeling deprived and mentally hungry. The result of much studying and soul searching gave me the knowledge and inspiration to create solutions for following 5 key topics.

Key 1
Covers childhood messages, environmental factors and customs that can override your attempt to lose weight. Examples: Eating all the food on your plate despite being full, or eating certain foods out of habit or custom. These messages need to be erased from your food voice to allow you to move on and lose weight permanently.

Key 2
Led me to research the neuroscience of eating and how the brain can control our food choices. Which food affects the brain, how the brain sends signals to eat, the fuel dictated by

the brain and how this influences food urges. I learnt how important is it to eat food I really enjoy as opposed to food choices I made only to lose weight. An example of this is not feeling satisfied even though your stomach is full, urging you to seek out food which has the feel good factor, resulting in over consumption of sugar and carbohydrate foods. How many times have we eaten a diet meal, felt full, followed by the most overpowering cravings? If they are too intense, we are compelled to eat. "**How do I take control?**" The answer to this question was for me the most incredible discovery I have made, as it has brought me peace of mind and balance. I now know my indulgence was nothing to do with my will power as sugar and carbohydrate affect the food voice negatively more than any other food. I do not hear this food now apart from the odd occasions.

Key 3

This key covers the fat burning and storage mechanism. You will learn how a high carbohydrate diet can cause insulin problems, turns the excess consumed into the following; **stored body fat, a fatty liver, high levels of fat in the blood (triglycerides) and faulty hunger and fullness signals.** I learnt, for example, that in order for my body to actually burn fat from stored cells it needs an adequate supply of water to enable this biological process. Yes, I know all diets say drink plenty of water, but I learnt **why**. There are many more facts that have amazed me whilst at the same time helping to put the missing pieces in the weight loss jigsaw together.

Key 4

Is the glue that connects all the keys together as beliefs form the basis of our actions. We cannot successfully change our actions if our beliefs are out of line. We will find many excuses to fail despite wanting to lose weight and keep it off. Our failures may be presented as outside events happening to us, but deep down we are responding to old limiting beliefs such as:

- Fear of change, fear of being hungry
- Fear of being deprived of certain foods
- Telling yourself you have a slow metabolism
- You are big boned or have always been large
- You life is too hectic
- It is your hormones
- You are over 40 and everyone has problems losing weight then
- Menopause or manopause causes stubborn weight gain.
- Your energy levels are low, but you put it down to age or lifestyle

Key 5

The diet programme explains in detail the best foods to eat in order to lose weight whilst improving your health and energy levels. This key includes:

- Carbohydrate, fat and protein, their role and benefit to your weight loss and energy levels.
- How much to eat in each category and why
- What food to avoid or limit, the reasons why are explained.

- Maintaining metabolism - why missing meals and not eating enough is a problem.
- How to cope with difficult situations such as eating out, holidays, stress and other life situations.
- How simple carbohydrates affect your food voice to the point where this food can be all you hear.
- The connection between fat storage, lack of energy and feel good chemicals in the brain.

The explanation of the first key will start in the past with a story, which will help you understand the history of how we learnt to eat junk food and how families acquired a taste for sugar in particular. Giving you a diet without you understanding the history will not work. You need to know how you have been programmed during childhood to eat certain food and the emotional connections you have developed. This is the first factor you need to address for long-term weight management. If you remain in the dark as to the core issue, you will not be in full control of a long lasting solution. The history of how our eating trends have evolved into our current junk food revolution is the first key to understanding how our brains have been programmed to eat in a certain way. The other four keys will enable you to finally unlock the weight loss door giving you access to new techniques to support new dietary changes.

"Give a man a fish and you feed him for a day. Teach a man to fish and you feed him for a lifetime." Buddha.

My aim is to teach you how to be in total control of your weight issues for the rest of your life. I want you to have the tools and the power to stop food taking control over you.

Most diet programs attack weight loss in a tip of the iceberg manner by ignoring the largest part of the problem hidden beneath the surface. The Food Voice Diet will teach you how to become the boss of your food intake for a lifetime.

KEY 1 HABITS AND ENVIRONMENT

The patterns of what and when we eat have developed since childhood as we have been influenced not only by our immediate family, but also by societies eating habits and trends. Each generation has its own trends, depending on many factors such as what food was available in the country, individual budgets and eating patterns.

As our food supply has become over abundant, it is now consumed without necessarily being connected to being hungry but for the taste, sensations and experience. What we currently choose to eat, or are compelled to eat, lies partly in our history.

LEARNT EATING BEHAVIOURS FROM CHILDHOOD EXAMPLES

- The types of food and drinks consumed
- How many meals per day including snacks?
- The size of your meals. How many helpings did you normally eat?
- How many times a day did you eat sugar and junk food?
- Your customs and traditions
- Trends and fashions

Our current generation is experiencing food mania as the result of the copious choices and quantities of food that have flooded the market place. The choice of foods available has become excessive and food has turned into an all day event in our lives. The most problematic food group affecting weight management is junk food.

WHAT IS JUNK FOOD

Junk food is a slang word for a class of processed food, which has little nutritional value and is generally high in fat, sugar, salt, additives, chemicals, preservatives and flavours. Junk food tends to be high in calories without satisfying hunger adequately. Junk food does however activate the brain to release chemicals called neurotransmitters that have similar effects to other substances such as alcohol and drugs. Junk food tastes good and it makes us feel happy temporarily. I will cover this subject in more detail later and fully explain why you can let yourself off the hook if you feel bad that you have not been able to rely on will power to lose weight in the past.

WHY WE LIKE JUNK FOOD

- Mood lifter. Feeling of a reward
- Stress and anxiety relief, comfort eating.
- Satisfies urges and cravings
- Something to look forward to eating
- Helps to promote denial of dealing with real issues, numbing of emotions
- Can be shared and enjoyed alone or in groups

- Socially acceptable
- Cheap to buy, the packaging adds to the product enjoyment.
- The taste and experience is good
- Improved self worth by buying food brands or eating in restaurants with a certain image
- Convenience and availability. Time saving, no cooking or washing up. Wanting more free time, not wanting to cook
- Familiar or similar foods to those eaten during childhood

NEGATIVES OF EATING JUNK FOODS

- Weight gain, toxin overload which the body struggles to process causing many side affects
- Regret and guilt
- Feeling helpless by choosing food over how you look and feel.
- Depression, sadness, discomfort, mood swings
- Health issues and future health risks, low level of well-being, lack of nutrients (malnutrition)
- Lack of energy, sluggishness, lethargy, poor concentration
- Undermines regular appetite management and portion control. Promotes hyper-eating.
- Failure to stick to diets
- Wasting money on junk food
- Clothes do not fit properly
- The amount consumed is increasing
- Withdrawal symptoms if not consumed
- Feeling out of control
- Tooth decay, weight related illnesses
- Calcium deficiency from carbonated beverages

- Addictions despite negative impact on health and life
- Makes digestion difficult due to synthetic ingredients and lack of fibre
- Does not satisfy appetite, easy to overeat.
- Metabolising high levels of sugar and starches strips our body of B vitamins, calcium, potassium, magnesium, enzymes.
- A negative food voice

Sugar and junk food deplete your vitamin, mineral and enzyme reserves.

Sugar may appear to give you energy in the short term but the long term use of sugar for energy depletes your vitality in the following way.

B vitamins are essential for the proper functioning of your nervous system, they are used up when you consume sugar and junk food. A lack of B vitamins causes many side effects such as anxiety, fatigue, stress, blood sugar problems, congestive heart failure, allergies, hair loss, skin problems and lack of neurotransmitters affecting mental health. Lack of B12 in particular, causes tiredness, exhaustion, weakness, depression, poor memory, anaemia

Mineral deficiency conditions include, asthma, low back pain, low blood sugar, diabetes, PMS and depression

Enzyme deficiency conditions include brain fog, mood swings, joint pain, digestive issues, insomnia, acid reflux and infections. **The Food Voice Diet helps to correct mineral, vitamin and enzyme deficiencies.**

HOW OUR BRAIN WAS TRAINED TO LIKE SUGAR...A STORY

Alice was born just after the war ended to loving parents who had experienced much hardship. They had been on rations for many years and had felt deprived of many of the foods they once enjoyed along with the rest of the nation. The post war diet consisted of mostly home grown, traditional food. The food supply although limited, was in fact healthy as there were no ready meals and fast foods for sale.

However, once rationing ended the nation celebrated in many ways and food was one of the main things that people looked forward to. The foods that were limited and much sought after were classed as "treats" and it was this type of food that Alice's mother rushed out to buy and prepare for her loved ones. The main treats came in the form of sweet foods such as sugar, which had been severely rationed. Giving sugar to family and friends was considered an act of love. The foods they enjoyed most were those they had been denied, such as cakes, jam, pie, chocolate, pastries and sugar drinks. Such was the celebration of having these foods that they became a real gift, something to look forward to as they now tasted even better. These treats were consumed happily and liberally as they represented the victory of the war and the rejoicing of having a normal life once again. Other sugar drinks such a fruit juice and soda started to become popular and Alice soon developed a taste for these drinks in preference to plain water.

Mother and father also loved sweet drinks and loved to heap teaspoons of sugar into their tea. Mother was anxious that Alice ate all her food as she was told that bigger babies were healthier. Alice was encouraged to eat as much as possible as her mother believed that a larger child was less likely to get sick. Relatives would often praise Alice for her weight and mother always felt proud when they did so. Thin children were considered malnourished and possibly from lower income households.

Alice was delighted with the treats and she soon learnt to love all of these foods and especially the feelings the foods brought to their home. Everyone in the house was very happy when mother made a cake or biscuits and this soon became Alice's favourite time of day. In the morning, Alice would have heaps of homemade jam on toast and was told, "what a lucky girl you are to have this food." Sometimes mother would say, "I will make you jam tarts today if you are good". Alice very soon associated sweet foods with love as mother gave these to make her happy. Father also loved the treats because they cheered him up when he came home from work. As he placed the food in his mouth, all that could be heard was a very long "mmmm", informing mother he was in heaven eating her delicious food. Every Sunday mother would serve roast dinner on the kitchen table and make a very special dessert that she always saved for the weekend. Alice always had second and sometimes third helpings and her proud parents frequently commented on her large appetite.

Adults frequently gave Alice sweets. During family visits she was always given a slice of cake, pie or a handful of toffees. There were no restrictions on the amount of sugar consumed as Alice's parents had no idea that excess sugar was not good for health and well-being.

As Alice grew up she was pleased to be able to buy sweets and candy in the local paper shop as her parents gave her pocket money once a week. She would run to the shop with her best friend, Patricia, who lived next door. Alice would choose her favourite hard-boiled sweets and Patricia would do the same, they would swap two sweets each, this made the treat even more fun. Each morning at school break, all the children were given a glass of milk along with two biscuits. School finished at 3pm and Alice would make the long walk home with Patricia, working up an appetite. Upon her arrival, mother would heap scoops of her homemade jam onto a slice of bread as a snack because Alice could not wait until dinner time. At bedtime, Alice would round off her day with a couple of biscuits and a glass of milk. The End

The moral of this story. Rationing improved the diet of the British population, as overall people ended the war fitter and healthier than they had ever been before, or have been since. This diet consisted predominantly of nourishing traditional foods. Food rationing in Britain lasted from 1940-1954. In 1946, bread was added to the ration list and sweet rationing was halved. Eating a healthy diet of simple home cooked natural foods improved health whilst introducing excess sugar in food and drinks had the opposite effect. Weight gain statistics have rocketed bearing testament to the fact that processed junk food is the main cause of weight issues to date.

FOOD SUPPLY CHANGES FROM 1946 TO CURRENT DAY

- Sugar consumption increased dramatically in both food and drinks
- Natural sugars were replaced by artificial and synthetic sweeteners such as high fructose corn syrup
- Natural animal fats were not recommended, processed manufactured vegetable oils were introduced
- High fibre whole grains were replaced by processed refined grains
- Natural flavours exchanged for artificial flavours
- Grass fed meat changed to cereal fed meat to fatten up animals faster to maximise on profits
- Manufactured processed food flooded the market place. Without perhaps realising we added to our diet preservatives, chemicals, processed fats, artificial flavours and colours, artificial sugars, synthetic vitamins and refined grains.

THE EFFECT ON WEIGHT AND HEALTH

The ingestion of so many processed food chemicals and additives, along with the increased consumption of sugar, introduces many toxins for our body to process and the effect of this strain can result in the following:

- Processing toxins and synthetic substances puts a strain on the liver and depletes vitamins, minerals and enzymes.
- Digestion problems, hormone imbalance.
- Weight gain especially around the middle

- Decrease in energy, increase in stress
- The pancreas produces more insulin than normal, leading to insulin resistance
- Fatty liver, high blood triglycerides (fat in the bloodstream)
- High levels of LDL (bad cholesterol)
- The body is unable to burn stored fat
- Increase in food cravings due to blood sugar fluctuations
- Hunger and fullness signals spiral out of control
- Lack of nutrients, malnourishment
- Reduction in brain chemicals affecting mental health
- A range of illnesses (see list from NHS and WHO)

The body starts to degenerate over time, which we shrug off in the beginning and justify our weight gain as an age or hormone issue and our tiredness is due to our hectic lifestyle. This slow erosion of our health and well-being lulls us into to thinking that feeling below par is our normal set point. We have no way of observing our insides which leaves us blind to the effects that food has on our internal organs. The communication between our internal and general health is via various symptoms such as how we look and feel. Excess weight is a message from the body that something is wrong with the way your body is processing the food you consume. Excess weight and a toxic diet can cause a further degeneration of your health along with continued weight gain. Our body works best on a diet based on foods that are as close to their natural source as possible. Also in the right proportions of protein, carbohydrate and fats to help balance our blood sugar and insulin release. Just because shops sell vast quantities of processed foods, ready meals and junk food, it does not mean they are the best choice of food to live on. If these foods were not so readily available we would experience weight loss utopia, but unfortunately, we are responsible for what we consume despite the abundance of junk food worldwide. The demand for sugar gave birth to the junk food and sugar empire that is wreaking havoc upon our waistlines and health.

The sugar treats were so popular in the post war era that manufacturers began making a wider variety of products which increased their profits. The nation rejoiced and celebrated the range of food choices now available to them as the spiral towards overeating the wrong foods began to escalate.

Can you imagine being in Alice's shoes and growing up in her environment where the only thing to look forward to was treats in the form of food? This habit was the reward she would unconsciously reach out to in order to feel good. The adults of this era did what they thought was best for their children, however the programming was well and truly set and unfortunately, as of today we are all a product of this learnt behaviour. Many of Alice's messages have been passed down to us forming the foundation for our food behaviour conditioning. After many years of an increased consumption of sugar Alice would have developed a modified food voice such as:

"What sweets shall I buy on Saturday"

"I wonder what cake mother has made today"

"I am having milk with sugar and biscuits for supper"

"When I get home, I am going to eat heaps of sugar sprinkled on bread"

"We have steamed sponge pudding every Friday it is my favourite"

"When I am hungry my first choice is always sweet food it makes me feel good"

THE POST WAR LESSONS

• Sugar is a cheap feel good food to be used liberally

• Sugar desserts are the ideal way to finish a meal. This quickly becomes a habit by repeated daily practise and will be fully ingrained in the unconscious choices and repeated behaviour patterns in adulthood.

• "Eat as much as you can and always finish all your food." This pattern programmes the child to override the feeling of fullness and to continue to eat regardless of the message to stop. After a while, the body no longer registers feeling full as the child learns to overeat. After rationing, parents remained anxious and continued with this advice out of love and what they thought was right at the time.

- Being chubby was viewed as healthy and a way to prevent sickness

- Children were given food to cheer them up or as an aid to discipline

- Sweet and manufactured foods were viewed as a sign of affluence

- There were no guidelines or government health information regarding sugar consumption

- Good home-makers baked for their families to show love and affection

- Eating sweet-based desserts were part of a balanced diet

- Big appetites were encouraged

- Sugary drinks were now available, the trend was set not only to eat sweet foods, but now the drinks contained sugar.

THE CURRENT DAY FOOD MESSAGES

- Children are still rewarded with sweets and junk food for being good

- Frequent TV commercials are shown to stimulate our brain to respond to desiring these products

- Television programmes show actors eating sugar and junk foods. This encourages people to copy what they see by influencing behaviour

- Junk food treat syndrome has hijacked the choice of food people make. "Why not treat yourself" thinking is overtaking healthy eating choices. Once a food is classed as a treat, we will want more

- Ready meals can be bought not cooked at home. Nutritional content is not as important as taste

- Unhealthy takeaway food has become part of a weekly routine in many homes

- Sweets and snacks are part of everyday life and no longer occasional foods

- School meals are mostly ready meals and junk food, as many schools have given into consumer demands

- Children may have some basic information about nutrition yet choose junk food out of habit, availability and fashion. Junk food can be cleverly disguised as healthy food to appeal to parents. Fortified breakfast cereals and fruit yogurts are examples of high sugar processed food

- Many more children at school are now overweight, which adds to social acceptance

- Parents are under pressure from their children to buy more junk food and sweets

- Junk food and sweets are considered trendy and a "must have" by many children and adults

- Soda and sweet drinks containing excess calories of sugar and additives are the norm

- Processed foods are eaten in excess

- Super-size portions in meals and drinks are new trends

- Assuming that junk food is harmless. Denial is a common process used to avoid making changes as it allows us to continue indulging. Food addiction and denial are often linked

- Health related food illnesses are now very common even in childhood as more and more children have diabetes and fatty liver

- We have been programmed to use unhealthy foods as a way of showing love and affection

FOOD VOICES OF TODAY

- "I fancy some crisps and a coke as dinner is not for a while yet"

- "That large bar of chocolate is my treat after dinner, that can go in my shopping trolley"

- "I am so looking forward to a cup of tea and cake when I get home it has been a long day"

- "The kids are driving me nuts I need to feel better, a biscuit will do the trick"

- "There is nothing good on TV, I am off to the kitchen to check out the fridge"

- "The super-size menu only costs a bit more, I may as well go for it"

- "I can't be bothered to cook I am ordering another take away"

- "I must go shopping tomorrow I am running low on biscuits and crisps"

- "Break time! Thank goodness I need another snack, I'm starving."

- "Pizza and cola? Sounds good but its not that filling, I will have the brownie too"

- "An orange juice and a sandwich will do for lunch today I am in a rush"

HOW THE PAST HAS AFFECTED OUR FUTURE

We are now the adults and children who have grown up with many of the inherited food foundations from the post war era. We have been brought up with this learnt behaviour passed down via our families and environment, creating the desire for sugar and junk food as treats. We have this information stored in our mind as habits, customs, unconscious patterns, preferences and automatic responses. It is difficult when our logical mind is aware of what we should be eating yet we have a built in habit, which has been imprinted into our system since childhood compelling us to eat unhealthy food.

In technical terms, what has happened to previous generations is that the brain's reward system to eat sugar and junk food has been continuously reinforced. This subject is covered in greater detail in the next key. Therefore, every time certain foods are consumed the brain releases certain neurotransmitters such as dopamine, which make us feel good. To repeat the same feeling, more of that particular food is required and this is how cravings and addictions are formed. Once the brain has become used to this pattern of food and brain reward programming, a tolerance to the food is built up where more food is needed to feel the same way. This is in fact very similar to drug and alcohol addiction when more of the substance is required to achieve the same height of satisfaction. Our reward system becomes blunt by continuously eating junk food and as a consequence, our brain demands larger quantities yet our level of enjoyment can be lowered.

For example, if you have a message imprinted since childhood, insisting that you always eat chocolate in the evening, or you always eat desserts after dinner, it is now a deep seated habit and the urge to repeat this message is so powerful because the feeling is controlled by both habit and your brain chemistry. If on the other hand you are repeating the same patterns of eating as you did as a child but you are overweight and miserable it is time to face the facts that this old habit is no longer working and needs replacing. Letting go is not easy, but it is certainly possible with the right information and the right plan. This diet will help you to move on and the only way that can happen is for you to take control and stop allowing food to control you, which can easily happen with certain food types.

Read the food message lists again and write down which food habits you have acquired in your upbringing that you would like to change. These issues are discussed in detail later in the book under solutions to key 1, but it would help to make a note of what affects you most of all. Work only on the main issues to a maximum of four.

KEY 2 HOW THE BRAIN CONTROLS YOUR FOOD VOICE

You are now aware from Key 1 that you have specific beliefs and patterns about eating certain food from your childhood, your culture and environment. Next, I will explain how eating sugar and junk food may have affected your brain in that it has come to depend and associate certain foods with chemical releases that make us feel good. This has further strengthened and boosted the patterns established since childhood. The inherent nature of our brain is hard-wired with reward pathways. The human brain requires a certain level of reward, pleasure and stimulation each day to function at its best and maintain a feeling of balance. We are motivated to seek out food because of this hard-wiring. Food connects to the reward and pleasure centres of our brain ensuring we survive. We have to eat! Dopamine is the main neurotransmitter released during the consumption of junk food, alcohol and drugs. Over time, more of these substances are required in order to get the same release of this chemical, promoting weight gain and addiction. Serotonin is the other major neurotransmitter, which is released upon consumption of sugar and carbohydrate. This can have a calming effect that can promote comfort eating and using food for stress management. To get the same affect more of the same foods need to be eaten causing more weight gain and dissatisfaction.

LACK OF REWARD AND PLEASURE

The Food Voice Diet ensures that you will have an adequate supply of positive, healthy and satisfying brain messages whilst losing weight. If we do not get the pleasure and stimulation we need we become reward deficient and in this state, we can experience a very loud food voice and the following symptoms:

- Cravings for sugar and carbohydrates in a desperate attempt to feel good.
- Excessive appetite and or the inability to stop thinking about food.
- Mood swings
- Lack of concentration, feeling agitated, unsettled
- Feeling weak and unwell.
- Temperature change feeling hot or cold
- Mental hunger even though you are full
- Overwhelming desire to eat immediately

In order to feel better our brain will send instructions to the body to resolve this deficiency. Brain chemistry is the main reason why you feel so bad on deprivation diets as the brain will send messages via the nervous system forcing us to change this state as quickly as possible. This normally comes in the form of cravings, urges, feeling shaky and unbalanced. To get rid of this feeling you have to eat. Sugar and simple carbohydrate are the most easily used fuel, hence the foods most commonly craved. If we do not experience pleasure from eating food which complements our reward system, the body will rebel at some point. Eating low fat food you do not really enjoy or any diet food you eat, which does not make you feel good, works for a short period of time for this reason. Binges are, in part, a result of depriving the brain of reward and pleasure foods. For a diet to work in the long-term food should be enjoyable, satisfying and meet your nutritional needs.

Eating junk food on a regular basis is not recommended in this programme, it sabotages weight control and health.

MISSING MEALS AND NOT EATING ENOUGH

Another feature of our survival mechanism is that we are predisposed to choose high calorie food, an instinct we cannot override or ignore. Our instinct is to choose the foods with the most calories to ensure we can survive by storing fat in order to thrive in lean times and famine. This rebellion also comes into play when we consume insufficient calories, our survival mechanism sends an alarm signal that we may be entering a starvation or famine situation and apart from feeling hungry or unbalanced, our metabolism will slow down to compensate for the loss, plus our energy output automatically shuts down. This comes in the form of feeling tired, lazy, unmotivated, wanting to stay at home and lethargy. In addition, your blood sugar will drop which can cause cravings and hunger, reaching out for a junk food snack or giving into a major binge. When you eat again your lowered metabolism will result in additional weight gain and fat storage. The trick is not to allow your body to raise the starvation alarm in the first place. The same applies with allowing yourself enough food in the day and not trying to cut so far back attempting to lose weight too fast. Remember your body needs enough food every day to be able to perform the job of keeping you healthy and centred. Too little food will affect your health, slow down your metabolism and leave you feeling tired, vulnerable to stress and mental imbalance. Eating too little does not satisfy your appetite and deprives you of enough energy to burn leaving you hungry and tired - the perfect environment for a carbohydrate controlled food voice.

WHY THE BODY NEEDS HEALTHY FOOD

If our food choices are dictated by our brain, we can be consuming foods that serve our brain chemicals instead of supplying our body with the correct nutrients to be able to carry out the various tasks required for good health. When we are overweight and only view food from the point of view of taste, we have urges, we experience cravings and our thoughts are overloaded by food sensations. Food has been separated from its real job as the key to health and survival. The main tasks our body needs food for are:

- Growth, repair and maintenance
- Regulate your heartbeat. (The heart prefers healthy fat as it's source of energy)
- Providing fuel for energy
- The brain needs food to work efficiently and for positive mental health
- Digestion, circulation, organ maintenance
- Breathing
- Protection from illness and disease
- Hormone production

If the food we supply ourselves prevents our body from doing these jobs our overall health system starts to malfunction, eroding our feeling of wellness and balance.

To ensure that your body carries out the above tasks, you are required to consume a diet which allows it to work at maximum efficiency. In return you will experience weight loss, extra energy and improved health

THE BRAIN RESPONSE TO TYPES OF FOOD

Food is one of the most important means of survival making it an ideal target for manufactures to design food that can influence our choices. Brain chemistry is one of the main reasons why we desire to eat certain food without feeling hungry. In effect, we are feeding our brain. If you feel addicted to eating junk food this is the reason why will power does not work for more than a short space of time. Feeding our brain is important, but we need to feed our body the right foods to support our health and choose foods to keep our brain happy, but not addicted.

The reward centres in our brain are stimulated most of all by the list below. Junk food is designed to ensure stimulation is maxed up to the highest level to allow manufacturers to control a higher share of your stomach. You will be able to identify with the preferred food types you are most attracted to. It is good to know what appeals to you, as this will help you choose new foods that satisfy you whilst avoiding junk food.

Sugar
The term used in manufacturing is "the bliss point." This ideal amount of sugar renders the user the maximum on the reward and pleasure meter. Sugar is addictive, it can blind-side the user into thinking this product is a harmless treat.

Fat
The term used here is "mouth feel" our brain hard-wiring seeks out calorie dense food to survive which is why eating triggers pleasure signals.

Salt
Flavour burst is the term used for salt as it lights up a taste tip at the front of the mouth that causes pleasure and we feel the urge to repeat the experience. Hence, the way we eat salted crisps as it is hard just to have one.

Meatiness
This is connected to the fat content and the pleasure we get from chewing.

Textures
Crunchy, chewy, soft, liquid. The correct texture can really help sell junk food, as we prefer products that enhance the food experience in our mouths.

Aroma
This can heighten the pleasure and the desire to eat.

Calorie density
The body prefers heavy calorie dense food, which is part of
our survival methodology,
and junk food satisfies this instinct

Sight
Seeing the food directly or indirectly via advertising can be
enough for the brain to release chemicals in anticipation of
receiving reward or pleasure. If you are addicted to junk food,
you will be more vulnerable to visual triggers.

Flavours
Food manufactures can create flavours to trick us into tasting
something that is not present. Flavours without ingredients
maximises profits and cheat us out of real food. Synthetic
flavours also play a part in the production of addictive foods.

In order to change your old patterns of eating this diet will
guide you by helping you make new choices consisting of
foods you really enjoy. The plan is to keep your good brain
chemicals active, which is such an important part of diet
success. Remember deprivation and will power do not work.
Write down what you like most to eat and try to group your
choices into the categories above, but exclude sugar. For
example you may love chewy and meaty such as spare ribs,
or salty smooth, such as cheese, or crunchy spicy food such
as stir fry or liquid soothing such as creamy milk and fresh
cream, or soft salty such as smoked salmon and cream cheese.

THE FOOD IN SUPERMARKETS TODAY

Food manufactures have devised and produced every conceivable sugar item and savoury snack we can possibly imagine. Every 'E' additive, colouring, preservative and stabilizer has been added to these products. Food has been bent so far out of shape from its original source producing tastes and textures to ensure we get addicted physically, emotionally, psychologically and any other format possible. Specialists in brain science are employed by manufactures to help to maximise the addictiveness of food. Since the war, the demand for convenience and processed food has provided food manufactures with the power to choose which foods are made available for society to consume. As more and more home-makers started to work, home cooking was on the decline whilst ready meals and convenience foods were on the incline. Manufacturers have maximised on this in a very unhealthy way by preying on the reward pathways in our brain.

Sugar and sugar enhancers are added to ready meals and most processed foods. Artificial sugar sweeteners like aspartame and saccharine can cause adverse health issues. Grains are processed, removing most of the fibre in order to extend the shelf life of the product. The cheapest fats are used in most processed foods, which are not the beneficial fats the body requires. Preservatives, colours and chemicals are added to food to make it look and taste better. These foods over stimulate the reward centres in the brain which is why we keep repeating the same behaviour despite experiencing the many negative effects of doing so. Junk food is hyper palatable to ensure our brain get the maximum hit in terms of reward and pleasure, this means you remain hooked and the manufactures sell more produce. They win at our expense!!

In addition to the physical addiction of these products, manufacturers and restaurant owners have used advertising to train us to associate the consumption of their products to be trendy, fashionable and cool. Therefore, we feel a sense of elevated acceptance, achievement and self-esteem connected to eating that particular food. Social acceptance and bonding via shared meals can encourage people to develop a taste for the wrong food without even being consciously aware they are doing so. For example, you can learn to like a fast food ready meal if this was the only place you met your friends once a week. You would eventually associate the food with the friends and you have built up a happy connection to this food.

Your brain would then add its own chemical reaction to the emotional connection by releasing chemicals to the brain reward centre that has been stimulated by the sugar, fat and salt it has just received in large amounts.

The occasional consumption of sweet or processed foods has now become the staple diet for many people and consumed on a very regular basis as these foods are prepared to be addictive. These products contain plenty of sugar, salt and fats to maximise the effect on the consumer and it works. Once addicted, people will continue to eat large amounts of these products because they are now controlled by their neurological system. Food is now frequently chosen for the taste over the nutritional value. This vicious cycle of dependence is a real trap, which anyone can fall into without knowing the dangers. We assume the food must be safe for us to eat as we go into shops to buy this produce. This is certainly a false sense of security that most people fail to recognise. Ignorance is not bliss in this instance as many people have suffered for years with weight gain related problems as they were unable to control their bad eating habits. If we picked up a packet of biscuits with a warning that said **"over consumption of this product can lead to food addiction and obesity, please eat in moderation"** we would view the product with more caution. If eating at certain fast food chains became venues for the unhealthy minority, I am sure many people would not wish to be associated with liking or being addicted to such food. In addition, there are types of junk food products which trick the brain into thinking the calories have vanished and therefore we can simply keep eating them without registering that we have had enough. The technical name is "vanishing calorific density" foods; these foods melt quickly in the mouth so be aware of these products and avoid them.

- Certain packets of crisps and pretzels
- Buttered and salted popcorn
- Soda drinks.

In addition to food, sugar drinks such as sodas and many fruit juices have very high sugar and chemical structures that help develop sugar addiction to junk foods. Once people get a taste for drinks containing sugar they will be more likely to choose them by the nature of their brain hard-wiring. Water then becomes less and less appealing to our taste buds. Sugar drinks have been cleverly marketed as an essential part of a fast food meal or snack. This ensures more sales and ties us into the pattern of choosing this drink instead of water. Our brain chemistry readily supports this.

We are the unsuspecting victims of addictive food and here we are today trying to figure out why it seems so hard to stop overeating the wrong foods. As a whole, there appears to be a large cloak of denial in society allowing these addictive foods to be sold without any health advice. On one hand, governments provide information about our health yet on the other hand allow addictive foods to flood the market place. Children are frequently targeted by manufactures, supermarkets and fast food chains advertising, as they can be easily manipulated. Once children become regular users of junk food they normally remain an ideal customer for life by the fact that the food causes physical dependency. Children especially love sugar; it has been proven that sugar is addictive to the brain. A tolerance to sugar is easily developed and more and more sugar is demanded by the body to feel normal. Withdrawal from sugar can cause symptoms such as agitation, anxiety, headaches, lack of concentration and general feelings of discomfort.

SNACKING THE NEW HABIT OF THE MILLENNIUM

Snacking is now a billion pound industry as we are encouraged to eat more and more food in between meals. Eating all the time (hyper-eating) is the new market for major food manufactures as a new trend has been established in eating behaviour. The snacking phenomenon has really taken off, as people no longer need to wait until mealtimes to eat or drink junk food products. This trend increases the intake of calories from food with very low nutritional value, creating additional bad eating habits and can cause excessive hunger despite the calories consumed. There is also some confusion about where the line should be drawn between a snack and a meal as certain low cost, fast food products retail as snacks, but contain the calories of a meal. Most people are looking for the cheapest snack with the maximum taste. Easy access to the product is important, as time and stress are major factors in most lifestyles. Snacking is not unhealthy unless it is too frequent and involves the wrong foods.

WHY MOST DIETS FAIL

As overeating the wrong foods and the habits of the nation's junk food consumption grew, health issues began to evolve due to weight gain. As the health effects of obesity escalated so did the availability of diet books giving people information on what to eat, when to eat, how much to eat. From zero information, nations are now overloaded with facts about food, calories, exercise, metabolic rate, hormones, will power and thyroid glands. We are now at the stage of information saturation point with facts and figures about what we should eat.

Diet books cover a huge range to suit all types of people's needs tastes, and health requirements. There are diet books for tots, teens, mums, dads, and the elderly. Health related diet books are available for people with diabetes, heart problems and many other health related issues. There are diet books for people who snack, the carbohydrate lover, the chocoholic, the meat lover, the vegetarian and the calorie counter. Of course there are diet groups, clubs and online diets all offering a wide range of solutions, yet the problems not only remain, but obesity is on the rise on a worldwide scale.

You have probably tried dieting and may have found, like many other people, that you managed to lose some weight, but then put it back on once your will power ran out of steam, which is normally sooner rather than later. The following is a list of the disadvantages of starting a diet, this may be very familiar to many readers.

THE NEGATIVE ASPECTS OF DIETING

- Failure to stick to the diet
- Not enjoying the food
- Hunger not satisfied.
- Feeling deprived, depression, mood swings
- The diet is not flexible or too complicated
- Inconvenient
- Not an enjoyable experience
- Stress, irritation, lack of focus and concentration.
- Feeling hungry and experiencing cravings
- Cooking separate meals for family or partner
- Lack of energy, lethargy, lack of motivation.
- Looking forward to breaking the diet
- Yo-yo dieting has made your metabolism too low to lose weight.
- Constantly thinking about all the forbidden food
- Loss of lean tissue and water not fat

With every diet, the end goal is to lose weight, however the result is that people go back to eating all the wrong foods again and put back the weight they lost and sometimes more. This is the unwritten chapter in the diet book to think, plan and dream about the end of the diet and all the foods you just cannot wait to eat again. This appears to be the message programmed into each failed dieter. When people announce they are "going on a diet" the plan is to lose weight, but deep down they are planning to deprive themselves of the food they really want for a while and then eat them again once some weight has been lost. Yes, there are the famous dieters seen on advertisements with their before and after photographs, but they are the minority and certainly not the majority. When we hear that obesity rates are increasing and that very soon 50% of the population will be obese, it gives the message diets do not work. Information about food and dieting will not help if you are programmed to eat for emotional and habitual reasons, as this will override any good intentions you have. If our brains have been trained to respond to feel good when certain food is eaten, when you try to deprive your brain, it will beat you hands down every time. If your carbohydrate consumption is too high, you may well be on a roller coaster of blood sugar swings, excessive hunger, cravings and fatigue, all stemming from this excess. Controlling certain foods like sugar is difficult for many people as "just one" leads to eating the whole packet because of our brain chemicals. Attempting control negotiations do not work with sugar, but what does work is switching to other healthier foods that **also** make you feel good. If you try to diet without building this into the equation, you will be back on the roller coaster once again with a food voice to drive you to distraction.

Sometimes the dread of going on a diet, despite being motivated to begin with, is all too much hence the start date is postponed. Failure can occur even before the diet has begun, especially for experienced dieters who have endured more setbacks. This is the reason why there are so many obese people; they simply decide to give up trying altogether and give in to eating without limits and controls. Remember is it not their fault, but the food they have been eating has weakened them into submission. Accepting how difficult it is to use willpower against certain foods give you the chance to find another way to win the war against the battle of the bulge.

WHY USING WILL POWER DOES NOT WORK

- Will power starts to weaken even after a few days on a diet
- Food cravings, urges and obsessions are stronger than willpower
- Watching other people eat junk foods
- Advertising
- Supermarkets prominently display junk foods
- Pressure from friends and family to indulge in non-diet foods
- A celebration or special occasion, can't enjoy social life
- Stress triggers, a desire to give into temptation
- Do not know what to do with spare time normally spent eating
- Feeling deprived.
- Hunger
- Lost some weight, allowing a reward.

- You knew you would give up before you started the diet, lack of self-belief.
- The end goal seems impossible or too much of a challenge or you have too much weight to lose
- Not really wanting to make permanent changes because you believe it is too hard
- Withdrawal symptoms from regular diet especially sugar and junk food.
- It's exhausting mentally and physically

LET GO OF GUILT FROM PAST DIET FAILURES

You must now be able to understand many of the reasons you have not been successful with weight loss on a permanent basis. It is important to accept that a considerable part of the problem is not related to your personal failure, as the battle against food is a bigger problem than simply your will power versus food. This battle is far larger than you realise, as it involves addictive food, childhood conditioning, insulin and fat storage issues and your faulty beliefs about food. There are more people and products against you than for you. Shopping can be a war zone as you can more often than not come home with more junk food items than you had planned to buy. You now know it is not simply that you are unable to control yourself-your brain has been hijacked by junk food because it gives you feel good rewards and pleasure. You have been programmed since childhood to enjoy these food, they were given to you to make you happy, stop your tears, and celebrate birthdays, Christmas and other special occasions. This problem has arrived on your doorstep over a long period of time, however the solution is available here right now.

Guilt has no place on this diet programme, hopefully you have experienced the big AH-HA moment and realized most of what has been happening to your waistline was out of your control or influenced by many other important factors. Stressing about weight is actually counter- productive to losing weight so keep your mind on your future weight loss goal and move forward. There is nothing wrong with your will power either under normal circumstances, but not against specific foods! The main focus is to learn the lesson and move on. On this eating plan, you will not have to go into such epic battles against food so read on ensuring you know all the facts concerning the reasons for weight gain. Do not skip to the diet section without reading the details as this diet information is vital to your long term success.

KEY 3 CARBOHYDRATES AND FAT STORAGE

Eating excess sugar and carbohydrates are stored as fat. There is a considerable amount of science in this key, but I will keep the facts as simple as possible. This will help you to understand why eating this food type has contributed to not only weight gain, but also cravings, lack of energy, excessive appetite and hunger. If you are eating too much sugar because of your childhood patterns from key 1 and your brain is dictating that it wants rewards and pleasure from sugar foods in key 2, then you will be choosing a diet based on a high intake of sugar. Many people are not aware of foods that turn to sugar when digested such as bread, pasta, rice, crackers, noodles, pastry and potatoes. These foods are called carbohydrates and provide energy for the body. The amount of fibre helps to slow down the sugar rush, which is why some carbohydrates affect the blood sugar rapidly versus a slow release. Sugar is hidden in numerous savoury processed foods such as soup, baked beans, sauces and ready meals, Sugar has over 40 different names in food manufacturing such as:

Sucrose, sugar, brown sugar, golden sugar, yellow sugar, invert sugar, grape sugar, date sugar, fruit sugar, beet sugar, fructose HFCS high fructose corn syrup, sorgurn syrup, malt syrup, golden syrup, carob syrup, fruit juice concentrate, fruit juice, xylose, lactose, cane crystals, glucose, glucose solids, agave nectar, dextrose corn sweetener, honey, molasses, maltose, maltodextrin, caramel. **Processed foods often contain various types of sugar, which helps to hide the grand total from the consumer.**

Sugars vary in levels of sweetness. High fructose corn syrup is the most commonly used sugar in food manufacturing and confectionery, as it is much sweeter and a cheap substitute for cane sugar produce.

Sugar	Relative Sweetness	Other Name
Sucrose	1	Sugar
Glucose	0.7	Grape Sugar
Fructose	1.1	Fruit Sugar
Lactose	0.4	Milk Sugar
Maltose	0.5	Malt Sugar

It is no accident that food labels have the smallest font size to put us off reading just how much sugar and additives are present. The easiest way to avoid this problem is to limit the amount of processed food you buy and read the labels. Manufactures can claim that there is no added sugar, which does not mean that sugar is not in the product. Many low fat products contain large amounts of sugar, but they can appear healthy as the buyer is focusing on low fat. High sugar intake is linked to fat storage so be aware that low fat in a product does not mean what you think it means. By cutting down on your sugar intake you will allow your body to adjust to keeping blood sugar steady in between meals. The aim is to burn fat instead of storing it. Eating excess sugar causes one of the most detrimental food voices enslaving you to a life of cravings and binges.

SUGAR SUBSTITUTES

These products are appealing if you are just counting calories, which can blind side you into assuming the product is healthy. These products are man-made and therefore contain many chemicals the body is not able to process. Basically the substitute sugar tricks the brain into thinking the product contains sugar and the body may well be fooled, but you are still training yourself to feed your need for sweetness. The food may taste sweet, but the price you will be paying for it is a chemical overload, which can clog up your system. Remember a healthy body burns fat more efficiently than an unhealthy body. Ask yourself what you believe about your need or desire for sugar? There may well be an old belief you need to clear up before you move forward. Remember how Alice developed the taste for sugar by the repetitive habits and traditions she experienced. Sugar and carbohydrates mixed with dietary fat is the worst combination of any food for weight gain. Adding sugar to fat allows us to consume larger portions of fat than singularly. For example it is difficult to eat a large amount of double cream or butter in its natural state, but if the same ingredients are mixed with sugar very large amounts can be consumed without the same discomfort.

INSULIN AND FAT STORAGE

- Insulin is a hormone produced by the pancreas. It is released when carbohydrates are consumed. Sugar and simple carbohydrates such as bread, pasta and rice cause high levels of insulin release which then drop down dramatically causing blood sugar levels to drop suddenly.
- Large insulin releases are called insulin spikes
- Insulin spikes result in excess carbohydrate being stored as fat and higher fat (triglycerides) in the blood
- When insulin spikes subside, blood sugar can drop quickly which make us feel hungry even though we have recently eaten. Constant hunger and irregular appetite can be the result of insulin spikes.
- The appetite regulating hormone is called **leptin,** the hunger stimulating hormone is called **ghrelin**. Excess carbohydrates affects both hormones adversely.
- Low blood sugar causes sugar and carbohydrate cravings forming a vicious cycle.
- If regular excess sugars flood the body repeatedly, fat remains in storage
- Large portions of food even healthy food can cause insulin spikes.
- Missing meals causes low blood sugar, alerting the body more fuel is required as stores are dangerously low. This can influence overeating during the next meal, eating the wrong foods and lower the metabolism. Low blood sugar forces the liver to release stored glucose to the bloodstream triggering insulin again.
- Insulin spikes can cause the fullness and hunger signals to stop working

- Insulin resistance can cause the onset of type 2 diabetes. Insulin is released, but not detected.
- Alcohol is liquid sugar.
- Coffee causes an adrenaline release, triggering stored fuel to be released from the liver raising blood sugar.
- Stress chemicals act in the same way as coffee on the stored glucose in the liver and insulin release
- Excess simple sugars and refined carbohydrates are stored as triglycerides which can be released into the blood. The body can produces fat from sugar (including alcohol) causing fatty liver.
- Insulin spikes can be avoided with the correct diet.
- Too much carbohydrate causes an overload on the body system, causing an energy drain instead of energy release.
- Insulin is the fat storage hormone, therefore, more insulin = more fat. This forms the basis for The Food Voice Diet, which reduces insulin by reducing carbohydrate foods.

There are only two ways for the body to gain fuel for energy.

- From food recently consumed. A moderate amount of fuel (glucose) can be stored in the liver and muscles, but only enough for one day. Excess is stored as fat in our fat cells.

- Via glycogen (the stored version of glucose) stored in the liver and fat cells. If the body is healthy and supported by the right diet it can use the fat cells as energy in between meals.

STORING FAT VERSUS BURNING FAT

The body knows when it has recently consumed excess carbohydrate from your junk food meal or snack by the amount of blood sugar, which is now available for the body to use. High levels of insulin are released to reduce elevated blood sugar. The body uses glucose for its immediate energy needs, fills up the liver and muscles, but any excess is stored in the fat cells. The body is programmed to store the extra fat for reserves due to our survival instinct. After an hour or two, when the immediate fuel has been used you will get the signal from your brain that your are hungry again as the large release of insulin dropped your blood sugar too low due to your high carbohydrate meal. You receive a signal to eat again as low blood sugar is a red alert to get food fast. Ideally, your body should now receive the message that no more food is needed as fat stores are full, but your leptin signals are not working. Your fat burning switch is off due to your insulin spike. You should now be burning fat for fuel and using the fat stores to keep you going until the next meal. Your brain cannot function without fuel, it sends you signals and symptoms that will force you to eat again when blood sugar drops after an insulin spike. The symptoms can become quite severe such as unbearable hunger, lack of concentration, weakness, and the jitters. Your first urge will be for carbohydrate food, which is the body's way of getting the instant energy from the quickest source possible. You will interpret this as cravings and urges and grab the most readily available high calorie food you can. The foods most sought after in an attempt to feel better fast are sugar and junk food. Not many people remain balanced enough in this state to make healthy choices. Therefore avoiding this problem is a must for anyone who is serious about losing weight. This loop of constant hunger and cravings is caused by an out of balance blood sugar, insulin and leptin response Further health issues can occur as the carbohydrate dependency spirals out of control. **The result is additional weight gain and metabolic disruption.** The Food Voice Diet breaks the cycle of carbohydrate dependence, insulin spikes and the imbalances that cause fat storage, excessive hunger and cravings.

KEY 4 CHANGING YOUR BELIEFS

Beliefs are thoughts that you have accepted at some point to be true, indeed some of your beliefs are based on fact, but others are not. Many food beliefs are imprinted in our mind over a period of time, this process is not always conscious, as we do not automatically notice an unhealthy belief when it is formed. Food beliefs form part of your food voice causing either a healthy or unhealthy message communication to the part of your brain where you make decisions about what to eat.

Beliefs can include.

- Your views
- Your ideas
- Your approach to life
- What you stand for. What you identify with.
- Your opinions and perceptions
- How you feel
- Your likes and dislikes.

WHERE DO OUR BELIEFS COME FROM

The majority of beliefs about food are learnt from other people such as:

- Parents, teachers, friends, family and acquaintances. Significant relationships can affect our beliefs, as we tend to believe people who have an influence on our lives.

- Many other beliefs come from our own perception of events, advertising and our personal interpretation of information. The negative beliefs we have about food, eating habits, and eating issues can be magnified by our spin on how we feel, which actually is not based on fact at all, but we believe our version to be true. We often accept a limiting belief and are our own judge and jury hence, case closed a negative belief is now in place.

Upgrading and changing beliefs which no longer work for you is an important step to help you lose weight. Following a diet plan will not work if you have a belief, which will sabotage your success. Part 2 of the book covers solutions to changing old beliefs in detail.

If you are finding it hard to access your beliefs, ask yourself some of the following questions:

- Identify the reasons why you have gained or are unable to lose weight
- Do you eat too much, if yes what type of food?
- How long have you been eating the trigger foods?
- Do you have any strong attachments to certain foods?
- When did you start to put on weight?
- How many times have you been on a diet?
- Reason for previous diet failures?
- What triggers affect your eating negatively?

NEGATIVE BELIEFS

- "I have a really slow metabolism"
- "I am big boned and have always been big, I am doomed to stay that way"
- "All my family are overweight"
- "It is too difficult to diet as I have to make separate meals for my family"
- "I never have time for breakfast or lunch "
- "I have a sweet tooth or I am a chocoholic which is why I can't resist"
- "I can't believe I can ever lose the weight and keep it off"
- "I am scared of letting go of certain foods I believe I need to get through the day"
- "My eating habits have been so bad for so long its pointless trying to change"
- "I am tired because of work or family demands"

The big question to ask yourself about your current belief is;

"Is this belief based on fact?"

The chances are that you will find that your belief it not based on actual concrete facts, but more a combination of what you have concluded. This premise then gives you the option to change based on the new information you have now accessed. It is simple once you have identified the belief and taken the time to have a mental spring-clean. As with Key 1, it will be helpful to make a note of the main beliefs which are causing your weight gain. It would is most effective to work with two or three beliefs at a time or you may only have a single area to focus on. Most people know their main weak areas regarding food and which time of the day they are most vulnerable to going off track. An unhealthy food voice attacks you when you are tired and vulnerable making evenings a difficult time for many dieters. Once your food voice has been tuned to support you, the evening snack attacks will subside because you will have dealt with the problem in advance as opposed to waiting for the battle to begin when you feel helpless and prone to temptation.

"Things do not change we change" Henry David Thoreau

KEY 5 THE DIET WHERE DOES YOUR FOOD VOICE COME FROM
FOOD TALKS!

Your food voice is directly related to the type of food you eat which alters the biology of your body by changing hormone messages, organ function, blood composition along with messages from the nervous system and brain. Fat cells are able to receive communications to release and store fat, but to get this communication working to your advantage you need to feed your body the right diet. You cannot feed your body junk food and expect your body to send messages to your fat cells saying "lets burn fat and become healthy" in the same way you can't turn on BBC1 and expect to watch a programme available on BBC2. If you want your body to perform a task for you, it will require certain foods to do that job. The food voice you hear relates to the food your body receives, it echoes back to you. Let me explain a little more.

Our blood system carries chemical messengers called hormones to our cells and organs enabling a wide range of communications between various parts of your body. Hormones link to specific organs by sending signals to get a certain job done. Insulin is a fat storage hormone secreted by the pancreas by receiving messages from the blood sugar to get to respond, especially when you eat large amounts of carbohydrates. In reverse, if blood sugar is too low for example, when we miss meals or get stressed a different hormone is released by the pancreas called glucagon. This message informs the liver than it needs to release stored glucose in order to raise blood sugar. Yes, the liver can release its own form of fuel into your system without you eating anything and without your consent. Excess carbohydrates are converted into fat by the liver triggering fat storage as opposed to fat burning.

Eating excess carbohydrate causes messages to your system for example: The pancreas shouts loudly to insulin "We have a huge sugar load here help, release the maximum insulin now as we don't want the blood sugar going sky high you know how dangerous that is." Insulin shouts to the fat cells "do not whatever you do release any stored fat in fact we are sending a major shipment over to you right now as we have an overload and we need to get this stored, quickly fill up your fat cells ASAP." Insulin did a great job, but perhaps went a little over the top and an hour later the blood sugar is too low and is heading for a dip. Your food voice then tells you to "get me a sugar fix now" you may also get some physical symptoms in the form of urges and cravings and the process starts all over again with a carbohydrate, insulin overload. This is how your food voice directly connects to the food you have recently consumed. If you eat a diet rich in sugar and junk food the echo you will hear is the message to eat more of the same food. You are in effect planting seeds in your body via the type of food you eat. If you want a crop which yields a lean healthy body with lots of energy then planting seeds from The Food Voice Diet list will deliver the correct results for you.

High insulin levels create "a must have sugar now" food voice. High levels of simple carbohydrate food effect insulin levels more than any other type of food. Tuning out the ability to hear the call of sugar food is the only way to resolve this food issue and the way forward is via a change in diet.

WHAT FUNCTIONS DO HORMONES CONTROL
(hormones are controlled by certain foods)

- Appetite
- Hunger
- Digestion
- Fat burning a hormone called hormone-sensitive lipase (insulin inhibits production)
- Reaction to stress
- Proper absorption of vitamins and minerals
- Blood sugar regulation and metabolism
- Energy release
- Body clock

The hormone message service begins to form the basis for your food voice and all roads lead back to what you are eating. A diet consisting of excess carbohydrate will radically alter your hormone functions, the effects being the messages you receive from your food voice will be along the lines of.

- "I feel a bit weak I need something sweet let me see what I have"
- "I cannot concentrate on this right now I am going to stop for a cup of coffee and cake"
- "I am hungry again already even though it's not long since I had breakfast"

- "I cannot stop thinking about the do-nuts in that shop down the road, I really want one"
- "I hope the kids have left some biscuits I really need something to keep me going."
- "Dinner was nice, but I have to have some chocolate or I will not be able to settle."
- "I will eat this cake now and be good again tomorrow." (But tomorrow never comes)
- "I will just eat one or two "(but the whole packet goes)
- "Work is stressing me out I need to stop right now for my chocolate bar and take a break"
- "I did not sleep well last night, I will eat something sweet to get me through the morning"
- "I slept well but I still feel tired and drained, I need some sugar."
- "My cupboards keep talking to me, it's driving me mad"

WHAT AFFECTS WEIGHT LOSS HORMONES
(Also affecting your food voice)

1. Nutrition
2. Regular meals
3. Excess carbohydrates.
4. Quantity of food
5. Food toxins
6. Exercise
7. Sleep
8. Stress
9. Water

In solutions to key 5, The Food Voice Diet is explained in detail giving you simple solutions to change your food voice whilst enjoying what you eat and not feeling deprived. Remember this is not a diet where you will be hungry, eating low fat food you do not like, staying home because you are on a complicated diet, eating separate food from the rest of your household. Each solution takes you one-step closer to your new healthy food voice.

YOUR NEW FOOD VOICE AIMS

- Active when you are hungry and quiet the rest of the day.
- Positive, making healthy suggestions to eat food your body needs that day
- Helpful, pointing out new foods to try, keeping your diet varied, ensuring a wide range of nutrients are consumed
- Keeps food portions in control
- Sends reminders to drink water
- Informs you that you are not really hungry, but bored or other
- Does not focus on food mistakes, but helps by not repeating them in the future
- Helps you choose food to obtain plenty of energy, allowing you to enjoy life to the max
- Helps you stay mentally balanced
- Prevents your cupboards and fridge talking to you negatively
- Enjoying natural foods that taste delicious

"Struggle ends where commitment begins" Sumner Davenport

MEASURING WAIST CIRCUMFERENCE

Your waist circumference provides a general guideline to determine if you are overweight. The Food Voice Diet recommends using this measurement for people who like to track their progress. Not all people wish to use actual measurements and prefer being guided on how their clothes fit or how they look and feel.

1. Using a tape measure without breathing in and in a standing position
2. Start at the top of hip bone which should be about level with your naval, bring the tape all the way around (or level with the belly button)
3. The tape should not be pulled tight
4. Repeat to make sure note down your start point
5. Measure before breakfast and always at the same time

RESULTS. This measurement can reveal how your weight is distributed and as a measure for weight related issues such as coronary heart disease, metabolic syndrome, including type 2 diabetes, impaired glucose intolerance (insulin resistance), high blood pressure, low levels of good cholesterol (HDL) high triglycerides (fat in the bloodstream)

Belt size and waist size can be very different if a belt is worn underneath the stomach area. It is important to ensure the tape measure is in the correct place.

PROGRESS. Your waist measurement is important to track your progress, as scales are not accurate in terms of lost inches. You may build muscle from exercise, which weighs more than fat, you may have lost inches, which do not show, on the scales.

	Ideal	Average	Too high
Women	Under 31.5 inches (80 cm)	1.5 – 35 inches (80 – 88 cm)	Over 35 inches (88 cm)
Men	Under 37 inches (94 cm)	37 – 40 inches (94 - 102 cm)	Over 40 inches (102 cm)

PART TWO

SOLUTIONS

KEYS 1-5

PART TWO SOLUTIONS KEYS 1-5

SOLUTIONS KEY 1 CHANGING CHILDHOOD PATTERNS

It will be beneficial for you to write down the main negative food messages you have received from your upbringing, from the following list called Typical Issues. This should not take more than five minutes of your time. Writing the problem down is an important step enabling you to focus on areas you need to work on for weight loss. Making notes helps you make conscious decisions to help identify the areas of weakness and conditioning you have not been previously aware of. If you try to keep the list in your head, you run the risk of forgetting what is important after one week. By highlighting your trigger areas, you will be in control of making new choices and decisions. It can be difficult to access a belief about certain food habits, but the belief is there, you just have to dig a little.

The Food Voice Diet is different to other diets as it works at a deeper level by peeling back the problem layers which have contributed to weight gain. This is not a quick fix diet leaving you with unresolved issues. By resolving each of the five areas represented in the keys 1-5 you will have attacked your weight issue from inside out. Making positive changes to your past beliefs gives you access to a bright new future in terms of how your food voice communicates with you. Once you eradicate the old messages you will find it so much easier to control food choices.

TYPICAL ISSUES

1. "I eat all the food on my plate whether I am hungry or not"
2. "I go back for second helpings despite being full"
3. "I feel bad throwing food away, I eat it all rather than waste it."
4. "I always feel like something sweet after a meal even if I am full"
5. "I buy myself sweets and chocolate as a treat"
6. "When I go out for a meal I use it as an opportunity to eat as much as I can."
7. "Weekend is my time for overeating."
8. "I eat watching TV at night to relax."
9. "I plan what junk food I am going to buy each day and visualise the future enjoyment of eating it."
10. "I feel panicky when I am running out of crisps and chocolate."

Let us have a closer look at each of the above examples and examine each negative food habit a little bit further. Here are some examples of childhood related beliefs and how to make the mental changes

1. "I eat all the food on my plate whether I am hungry or not." This belief is often taught during childhood whereby now, not finishing the food makes you feel wrong or incomplete. Fear of being hungry can be connected to this belief generating anxiety and unease. Some people hate to waste food and would rather eat the food than be seen to throw it away. Adults sometimes eat the left over food on their child's plate when they have

this belief

NEW BELIEF: "I no longer need to eat all the food on my plate, it is causing problems with my weight, however, I do not want to waste food. I could serve smaller portions and use the leftovers tomorrow as I feel over full and regret my actions. I will learn what is enough to avoid being hungry later, if I am, I know that I have access to more food. My parents taught this to me out of love, they had learnt this from their parents who must have been worried where the next meal was coming from. My life is different, I have enough to eat on a regular basis. I can put one or two spoonfuls less on my plate. I can let go of my fear of being hungry or not having enough."

2. "I go back for second helpings despite being full. I remember doing this as a child because I had a big appetite and enjoyed my food. I am still doing this as I got used to second helpings, but now I am putting on so much weight and do not feel good when I am too full."

    NEW BELIEF: " I can always eat again later. I can slow down the speed at which I eat in order to remain in control. If I eat more slowly I will feel the signal that I am full. I can really enjoy my food without over filling myself. I will not be missing out or feeling deprived and I allow myself permission to change."

3. "I feel bad throwing food away. I eat this food to avoid wasting it. I am currently wearing this excess food on my hips. I need to sort this out in my head."

    NEW BELIEF: "I am not a rubbish bin, I will have more

respect for my body. My parents taught me not to waste food and they are right. I can freeze excess food if it is getting close to the sell by date. I prefer to be slimmer. I check sell by dates more carefully now when I am shopping by selecting items at the back of the display which last longer."

4. "I always want something sweet after a meal even though I am full. I was brought up this way. I like desserts, we always had desserts when I was young, but this habit is making me fat and unhappy now I am an adult."

   NEW BELIEF: "I do not have to eat food that causes weight gain, there are healthy desserts that I can really enjoy. I do not have to eat dessert to be happy if I choose foods that I feel are a treat, but don't include sugar. This way I give myself a reward without adding to my waistline."

5. "I buy myself sweets and chocolate as a treat. I spent my childhood doing this and have carried on because I look forward to it even though I am overweight and unhappy. I still want to buy these items as I they cheer me up, I can't seem to pass a supermarket check-out without buying something."

   NEW BELIEF: "I am not a child anymore and my body is not coping with the sugar. I will not feel deprived by letting go of this old belief as I can look forward to indulging in something else I really like, such as hot milk with melted dark chocolate topped with a teaspoon of double cream."

6. "When I go out for a meal, I use it as an opportunity
   to eat as much as I can. Eating out has always been an
   occasion to really let go and binge. I make the most of
   not having to cook and I eat different food. I accept that
   I am going out more than I used to which means that I
   am overeating more often than not. The results are not
   good, I am gaining more weight and when I look in the
   mirror, I cringe because I do not like what I see and wish
   I had not eaten so much. This feeling can last until I
   finally get to sleep, promising myself that next time will
   be different."

   New Belief: "Going out for a meal and overeating is no
   longer a treat if I am abusing my body. I now reclassify
   going out for a meal as a treat only because I do not
   have to cook and it is an enjoyable social experience.
   Overeating does not have to be included in the equation."

7. "Weekends are my time for overeating. I learnt this
   pattern as a child as both my parents worked so weekends
   were time to let go and enjoy lots of food. I associate
   weekends with TV snacks, big meals and desserts.
   Weekend blow-outs are taking their toll because I am
   getting bigger and bigger. I am less inclined to socialise
   because I do not feel good about myself. I do not want to
   be seen out as most of my clothes no longer fit."

   NEW BELIEF: "I can still eat well at weekends, enjoying
   food I do not have time to prepare during the week, but
   I can choose different, healthier food that I like. When

I think about it, junk food is not the only food I really enjoy. I can make some adjustments so long as I have food treats to look forward to at the weekend. I know that once I lose weight I will feel like going out again and food will not be my only focus at the weekend."

8. "I eat watching TV at night to relax. I always did this as a child because it was the best time of the day. My family made a big deal out of these nights and it felt special. I have come to associate TV time with snack time and find it relaxing, but later I feel guilty and regret it because I end up eating more than I wanted to. I know I can find another way to relax, eating is not the answer."

NEW BELIEF: "I can learn to swap junk food for other food. If I have a nice long bath and change into my lounge-wear, I will switch off and relax, I will then feel more like eating healthy food as opposed to junk food. I accept that eating extra food for stress relief does not work. My short term plan is to divide my evening meal, saving some food to snack on whilst I watch TV."

9. "I plan what junk food I am going to buy and visualise myself eating it throughout the day. I am not even sure when I developed this particular habit, but it seems to be getting out of control as I am thinking about this food a lot more. The anticipation of eating is taking up a lot of my head-space and I seem to think of it as the end goal of the day, as my treat. The trouble is I am putting on weight so fast and because this is upsetting me, I start thinking about cheering myself up with the food I know I should not eat."

NEW BELIEF: "I need something to look forward to each day which is not going to make me fat. There are foods that I can choose, and that I really like, which are not junk food. I can also look at planning other treats to look forward to, which do not cost a lot as I am on a budget. I know I can look after myself a lot better instead of using food which is not working."

10. "Junk food is addictive and harmful to health if eaten on a regular basis. I know I have been kidding myself that I can control buying these foods, but most of the time I end up overeating them and the more I have, the more I want. I accept these foods are produced to condition my thinking this way and if I keep choosing junk food, I am accepting all the negative effects they have on my body."

NEW BELIEF: "I can really enjoy food that is not junk food without feeling deprived. There is a huge variety of healthier options that will satisfy me, without opting for food with no nutritional value. I have so much to gain from making these changes and I now accept that junk food and weight loss do not go together. Junk food adds extra toxins, which my body finds hard to process, making me fat and draining my energy. The trade off for my new food treats is perfectly acceptable."

SOLUTIONS KEY 2 ELIMINATING ADDICTIVE FOOD

In Key 2, you learnt how certain foods take control of your food voice leaving you with suggestions that sabotage weight loss. The plan now is to take your power back from addictive foods and reclaim a food voice which works for you. The seduction of sugar and junk food lulls us into a false sense of security believing that the food is harmless and that we are merely indulging in a treat. This is where we are taken down the weight gain path, allowing us to form seriously difficult food habits which need to be pulled out of our thought process like weeds.

The list of foods on the charts at the back of this book cover a wide range of delicious foods supporting weight loss and boosting energy levels. It is time to look at this list and make a selection of the food you absolutely love to eat. In the diet section solutions key 5, you will find breakfast menus, cooking suggestions for lunch, dinner and lots of tips to help you fine-tune the foods YOU prefer to eat. The Food Voice Diet has avoided making a 7-day or monthly menu as it is of vital importance that you eat food you love, enhancing feelings of well-being. It is important that you meet the following requirements when making food choices

- Choosing food that satisfies the reward centre in your brain
- Really enjoying what you eat. Choose foods you look forward to eating
- Do not eat low fat versions of food you like which compromise taste
- Your mental happiness is important for successful and permanent weight loss
- Avoid foods that are potentially addictive, give yourself a fighting chance to succeed
- Make sure you eat a good breakfast with healthy fat to feed your body and brain
- Re-connect with the sheer joy of eating food that supports you in every way.
- Eating enough food and do not miss meals.

THE FINANCIAL COST OF EATING JUNK FOOD

Bad habits generally come at a cost, overeating not only affects you personally, but financially. The foods that are making you overweight involve a financial outlay as extra fat has not come free. In the next section we will cover the amount of money involved, how to use the funds you will save on better food choices to support your weight loss food voice. With the financial crisis fully underway it is time to be aware of the full extent of the financial cost of being overweight. I will cover the cost to your health later.

Once you calculate the cost of putting on weight and maintaining it, you can then make a decision on whether you really want to spend that amount and if you are getting value for your money. Are you happy? Have you invested well?

What do you have to show (or not want to show) for all the money you have spent and may continue to spend? Do you also spend this money helping family members develop the same spending habits? Alternatively, if you are not a parent yet what will the future spending be for your family based on your current food choices?

Once you have started The Food Voice Diet you will find you will respond differently to the messages that you may still get from your brain from time to time regarding old programming. In future these messages will be interrupted by your knowledge that certain food is addictive and can really set you back as you will recall how unhappy this food made you in the past. If you are in balance and feeling good, you will react differently to food triggers. Of course, there are times, when you may eat this type of food on certain occasions, as it would be almost impossible never to consume junk food again. Junk food can be inexpensive per item but it does not satisfy hunger adequately, other similar items are then consumed making the total outlay each day rather costly indeed. The mindset changes when it comes to buying junk food as we tend to justify this as a treat and not include it in the weekly food budget. An example of this mindset is complaining about the cost of real food but not the money spent on treats which light up the brain's reward centre. This is how brain chemicals lead us into addictive food habits and excessive expenditure on a pastime which is making us fat.

With the economy as it is the cheap and accessible treats are even more appealing as an affordable way to offer a reward to you and your family. For £1.00 or less, you can buy a junk food item. £1.00 is not a huge expenditure, it is so easy to talk yourself into spending a pound.

Let us now look at the real financial costs of junk food consumption
EXAMPLE: 1 treat per day for one person. Let us take a bar of chocolate, packet of crisps, a do-nut or a pastry at an approximate cost of £1.00 per day, or £7.00 per week, or £28.00 per month. The total spend per year is £365.00

The expense of one junk food item per day costs £365.00 per year and the result of this habit is shown in excess weight. If continued, which is often the case with addictive food; the habit will increase to perhaps two items per day, costing £730 per year! Your weight will, of course, increase in line with the extra food that you eat. The questions we need to ask ourselves are:

1.   Has spending £365 or £730 been worth it? What do I have to show for spending this money?
2.   How much weight have I put on in that year?
3.   What else could I have bought with the money?

Let us take another example using a family of four eating one item per day each.
For a family of four the annual cost is £1460.00
For one couple eating three items per day each the cost is £2, 190 per year.

My figures are more than likely conservative, as generally people will be spending more on substances that have no nutritional value, are making them unhappy, unhealthy and overweight. I am sure by now that you agree that your money can be better spent rather than buying food that makes you fat. If it is a complete waste of your money, time, energy, health and joy in life, you can make changes. The good part is now you get to decide how you would like to spend this money from now on. In order to be able to change your food voice urging you to eat junk food, it is of vital importance that you follow the steps in this book to ensure that you are successful. Will power does not work against addictive food.

EATING FOR BRAIN NUTRITION AND IMPROVED MENTAL HEALTH

The Food Voice Diet evolved from researching the nutritional data of certain food which supports the brain such as: **brain function, adequate energy, positive brain chemistry, mental performance and better mood control.** Sugar prevents brain cells from firing normally, affecting moods and other brain cell functions. The Food Voice Diet helps you make better food choices to support your brain and your taste buds.

Lack of adequate brain nutrition has been linked to the following; depression, bi-polar disorder, dementia, Alzheimer's disease, insomnia, brain fog, confusion, lack of concentration, bad memory, impaired learning ability, brain performance.

BRAIN FOODS

- Blueberries and other berries
- Wild salmon, tuna and other oily fish
- Nuts, seeds, fresh herbs and vegetables
- Avocados
- Healthy fats to carry vitamins A, D, E and K such as coconut oil
- Meat (with fatty edge)
- Poultry (with skin)
- Butter on cooked vegetables to aid nutrient absorption
- Dairy products if tolerated
- Home-made beef and chicken bone broths
- Dark chocolate and cocoa
- Bullet proof coffee (see breakfast menu recipe)
- Cod liver oil
- Organic barley grass

Remember, sugar and excess simple carbohydrates deplete your B vitamins, minerals and enzymes.

FINDING NEW FOOD TREATS

To avoid falling back into the mode of classing junk food and sugar as treats in order to give your brain a boost of feel good neurotransmitters, it is vital to find alternative foods which will also satisfy the reward pathway in your brain. The Food Voice Diet incorporates good brain chemistry as part of the philosophy of eating to help you retrain your food voice permanently. It is not possible to use sugar and junk food as treats due to the addictive nature of this food plus the effect it has on your blood sugar, insulin, satiety and appetite imbalance. Making your list of the most pleasurable food is very personal as what can send one person into food heaven is distasteful for another. In Key 2, you will find a list the food manufactures use to satisfy the brain chemicals to gain customer satisfaction, this includes textures, meatiness, mouth feel and flavour burst. Since I have reconnected with my new food treats, my old favourites no longer appeal to me and are just a distant memory of foods I once craved.

EXAMPLES OF NEW FOOD TREATS

- "I love the meatiness and chewiness of spare ribs and I savour the meat off the bones"
- "The saltiness of bacon dipped into a runny egg gets me out of bed in a heartbeat"
- "I look forward to a melted Cheshire cheese omelette which will make me totally full and satisfied"
- "There is nothing like a sumptuous rare steak with a bit of tasty fat, it works for me every time"
- "A spicy, crunchy stir fry with fresh green chillies makes my heart sing"
- "Hot milk with a cube of melting dark chocolate is my favourite comfort drink"
- "Roast pork with crackling, is a gift from the gods, it certainly goes on my treat list."
- "My weekend treat is a coconut pancake with bacon and a mug of bullet proof coffee; it just doesn't get any better than that for me"
- "Smoked salmon and cream cheese is the combination to die for. I love the perfect blend of flavour and texture"

- "Anything with fresh cream sets my taste buds alight and satisfies my soul"
- "Guacamole and hot toasted pita bread, ticks all the right boxes on my treat list"
- "Hot prawns dipped in garlic butter would be my desert island choice"
- "Satay chicken just out of the oven and sat on my plate is on my wish list"
- "The aroma of a Sunday roast wafting around the house fills me with a feel good factor from head to toe"

SOLUTIONS KEY 3 AVOID INSULIN SPIKES AND FAT STORAGE

Overeating carbohydrate foods especially in the processed format causes a rise in blood sugar and insulin. As the body struggles to deal with the overload, it has to store excess fuel as fat because there is limited storage space in the liver and muscles. If this process is frequently repeated our cells and organs become tired and start to lose the ability to work well. The insulin receptors become inefficient resulting in an even higher insulin release, which then lowers the blood sugar too much and we receive the faulty signal to eat again. In addition our fullness and hunger signals are also knocked out of sync. Also the liver can start to release too much fat into the blood stream and attempts to store more fat itself, which causes a fatty liver. Excess carbohydrate (including alcohol) can cause excess storage in our fat cells, a fatty liver and high levels of blood triglycerides even on a low fat diet, of which many people are not aware. The main function of triglycerides is as a stored source of energy, but in excess along with cholesterol, too much is bad for the heart, liver and weight issues.

Remember more insulin = more fat.

DANGER OF HIGH TRIGLYCERIDES
(Excess fat in the blood stream)

1. Raises the risk of heart disease and stroke
2. High blood pressure
3. High blood sugar
4. Diabetes 2
5. Obesity
6. Kidney disease
7. Under-active thyroid
8. High levels of bad cholesterol

The above illnesses can be controlled by a healthy diet in combination with weight loss. This is a catch 22 problem as excess hunger and the drive for high carbohydrate foods throw this faulty system even more out of balance. It is necessary to keep insulin and blood sugar low and, of course, limit unhealthy trans fats and toxic food in the diet.

CHOLESTEROL

Is a saturated fat, which circulates in the bloodstream, it is essential for many bodily functions, however it differs from triglycerides which provide energy for the body. The majority of blood cholesterol is made by the liver with a smaller amount from fat food sources. The two types of cholesterol are HDL the good type and LDL the type that causes clogged arteries and high blood pressure especially when the particles reduce in size.

ROLE OF CHOLESTEROL

1. Assists in the production of the outer cell wall
2. Creates bile to digest food in the intestines and helps to absorb vitamins A, D, E, K
3. Allows the body to make vitamin D from sunlight, necessary for good bones and teeth
4. Helps to retain salt and water
5. Production of hormones especially oestrogen and testosterone.
6. Synapse formation in the brain, helping you to think, learn and remember
7. Plays a role in building muscle and wards off infections.
8. Helps cell communication and regulates body temperature
9. Protein metabolism
10. Cholesterol can help the production of serotonin, a hormone helping to regulate moods
11. Brain tissue is made from cholesterol and saturated fat.

HIGH CARBS AND CHOLESTEROL

The majority of cholesterol is made in the body (up to 85%). What causes excess production? Excess carbohydrates cause insulin spikes which result in higher levels of triglycerides and **LDL cholesterol**. Refined carbohydrates, simple sugars and junk food are the main cause of insulin spikes. The liver converts this food into fat, the danger of course being, that the rate at which the liver is producing the quantity of fat spirals out of control. Therefore excess cholesterol is reduced by limiting simple carbohydrates which can cause cholesterol issues.

TIPS FOR KEEPING INSULIN LEVELS BALANCED

1. To avoid going into fat storage mode, never eat carbohydrate foods as a main meal or snack without protein. Avoid processed and ready meals, junk food and limit the amount of toxins in your food to keep your system healthy. Eat only complex carbohydrates.
2. Eat more protein and fat than carbs at each meal. This will help you to feel more satisfied after eating, control your blood sugar and balance out your appetite.
3. Add vegetables, not only are they good for you, but they add fibre to your meal which also slows down the effects of insulin.
4. All calories are not equal with regard to weight gain. For example, if you ate a normal amount of calories a day, but your calories were mainly all carbs you enter fat storage as the carbs turn to sugar and cause insulin spikes. If you ate the same calories in The Food Voice style of eating, you would use food as energy and be able to rely on your fat stores in between meals and lose weight.
5. Do not overeat, even healthy food, to the point of being overfull as this can also cause insulin spikes. For example if you get the right ratio of protein to carbs plus your vegetables, but ate a gigantic meal, you would have consumed an extra large portion of carbs and food that can create fat storage.

6. Eat regular meals, as missing meals can cause fat storage. Eat enough food.
7. Dehydration can mirror the signals of hunger. Make sure you drink plenty of water as this helps to fight fatigue by carrying oxygen around the body
8. Lack of sleep can cause your body to send you messages that you need carbohydrates or that you are hungrier than you think, in an unconscious attempt to get extra energy to cope.
9. Stress releases chemicals, which alert our system of impending danger, stress hormones are released along with insulin to help you have extra energy and fuel to deal with the issue. In addition to life in general, being unhealthy can cause stress. Stress can make you hungry. Getting your weight under control and feeling healthy, promotes resilience to other stress factors.
10. Reduce coffee and caffeine intake as these drinks can cause stress hormone release affecting blood sugar and insulin release.
11. Eat healthy fats not processed and manufactured such as margarine and vegetable oil.
12. Moderate exercise
13. Limit alcohol consumption and consume with food not on an empty stomach.

EXCESS STRESS CAN AFFECT WEIGHT LOSS

1. Some stress is good for us as it helps us to function and survive as well as giving us the push we need for achievement and improvements. In excess stress can have negative effects on our ability to lose weight and remain

on a diet. Our fat burning mechanism is affected by stress. Losing weight will considerably lower your general daily stress quota helping you find balance once again. The Food Voice Diet promotes nutrient rich food and supplements to further reduce the internal stress caused by a bad diet.

2. Being over weight can cause stress stemming from negative feelings such as low self-esteem, a limited lifestyle, lack of confidence and similar issues. This affects our body, mind and spirit.

3. Eating a bad diet, which lacks the correct nutrients to support our body functions, can cause stress on the physical body. If the body is unhealthy it will not function as well, thus fat burning can be impaired.

4. Bad health causes worries, fear and stress. Feeling healthy helps us build strength to be able to deal with illness more effectively.

5. Physical pain causes stress. Improving your diet promotes healing

6. Stress affects how hungry we are, how much we eat, the type of food we eat and in this state, the food choices we make are not the best.

7. Stress causes a release of adrenalin that instructs the body that we need more fuel to deal with the problem as cortisol the stress hormone is released. The liver then releases glucose from its store into the blood stream followed by an insulin response to the increase in blood sugar. During this process, fat burning is switched off and fat storage turned on. Insulin resistance can result in high levels of long-term stress effects on the body.

8. Belly fat (visceral fat) contains receptors for the transmission of cortisol the stress hormone. The larger this area is, the more predisposed you are to excess stress.
9. Constant stress can affect the thyroid gland, which controls your metabolic rate.
10. Reducing stress helps to build muscle and tone up
11. Stress reduces the production of feel good hormones such as serotonin

THE FOOD VOICE DIET STRESS TIPS

- Eliminate extra toxins from foods that are weakening the body. This is something you can do immediately and easily make these changes.
- Drink at least 10 glasses of water a day.
- Follow The Food Voice Diet to keep you strong, healthy and positive.
- Obesity related health issues are preventable.
- Set a goal to start this diet plan today.
- Work on the beliefs you want to change to ensure you lose weight
- Let go of the past and commit to this programme, now you finally have the information you need to succeed. Do not stress about the past you cannot change it.
- Congratulate yourself on the new information you now have at your disposal in this book. Knowledge is power.
- Make a plan or plan to fail. Complete the steps 1-14 at the back of the book
- You will have a list of food treats chosen by you that will ensure you will not feel deprived. This is often one of the main fears causing anxiety about dieting.

- Give this new diet programme a chance without feeling stressed about making a change. Have a "bring it on" attitude and take a brave step forward.
- Get enough sleep as lack of sleep causes stress triggering food cravings and excess carb consumption.
- Do not over exercise as this can cause stress to the body.
- Be prepared, stock up on groceries for home cooking, short cuts for meals in a rush, to avoid going off track.
- Make YOU a priority–put your weight and health on the top of your list of priorities.
- Taking action as opposed to putting something off can shift stress very quickly.
- When stress does occur, ask yourself if what ever or who ever is stressing you is worth it? Remind yourself that stress causes weight gain motivating you to work on solutions.

THE FOOD VOICE DIET ENERGY TIPS

Having plenty of energy is essential for enjoying your life and making the most of each day. There is no point losing weight only to feel exhausted, bad tempered and unhealthy. Relying on caffeine and sugar for energy is a sure sign that your diet needs to change. If this is how you have been getting through most days accept that this is not genuine vitality as you can easily crash and be left depleted and exhausted.

- Lose weight
- Follow The Food Voice Diet plan (Excess carbohydrate causes energy blocks)

- Excess sugar uses up your B vitamins, minerals and enzymes causing fatigue
- Eat breakfast (see Key 5) Start the day with coconut oil bullet proof coffee
- Use mostly coconut oil for cooking,
- Take barley grass twice a day
- Take cod liver oil in the morning
- Drink enough water
- Moderate exercise 3 times a week for 10-20 minutes to start with.
- Stress reduction, stress drains your energy reserves. Focus on solutions not problems.
- Adequate sleep
- Limit alcohol and caffeine.
- Take a shower or bath
- Sing, dance and laugh as much as possible. Count your blessings.
- Meditate or power nap
- Get organised. Left over jobs drain your energy reserves.
- Spend time outdoors when you can (especially barefoot)
- Learn something new, find a new hobby, stimulate your mind.
- Do not compare yourself to other people just focus on your own improvements as that's what counts.
- Keep positive and do not give up on your weight loss goal and improving your health in as many ways as possible. Every small improvement counts.

SOLUTIONS KEY 4 CHANGING OLD BELIEFS

The beliefs we have about our body image, dieting, what to eat and when to eat, can form the basis for the internal conversations we all have with ourselves on a daily basis regarding food. Your food voice can be positive or negative, but with weight gain issues there is more of a negative voice barking orders, which unfortunately stems from this imbalance. The beliefs we have form our own voice instruction manual, which we follow until we change the content. In order to change a belief, first identify it and then challenge that belief. Changing a belief is like a personal permission slip to re-programme your instruction manual. The food voice will still be communicating with you in your head, but it will be following your new orders.

THE FOOD VOICE

Is a message service programmed by our beliefs and our body chemistry. The healthier your body combined with positive food beliefs, the more peace and harmony you will experience. Your food voice can run all day without any breaks if your body is out of balance, experiencing cravings and food addictions. The food voice can hugely influence the type of food you choose, leading to further weight gain. The aim of this diet programme is to tune your food voice to the fat burning version designed to help you lose weight and is only active at certain times in the day. This will allow you to get on with other tasks and enjoy your life.

YOUR POSITIVE FOOD VOICE

1. Helps you make the right food choices
2. Directs you to foods which make you feel good in a healthy way
3. Leaves you in peace outside of meal times
4. Negotiates difficult decisions with you. You can weigh up the pros and cons of choices and look at options
5. Points out foods your body needs depending on how you are feeling and your body's requirements
6. Gives you clues when you are out of balance as to what else or who else is bothering you.
7. Motivates you.
8. Helps you boost energy levels
9. Promotes weight loss

THE NEGATIVE FOOD VOICE

1. Is not reliable
2. Has two messages, eat the wrong food and eat too much.
3. Does not switch off in between meals
4. It wants constant attention and to be the solution to all life's challenges and issues
5. There is no on and off switch or volume control.
6. Can be voiced over by addictive food types where the food is controlling your choices not you
7. Drains your energy, de-motivates you, helps you resist positive change.
8. Wants you to waste your money on addictive foods

PERSONAL BELIEFS

Personal beliefs tend to have emotional content as we have normally arrived at that particular belief via a negative experience which has often been upsetting. During negative states, when feeling vulnerable, it is easier to believe something if we are not in the right frame of mind to question our thoughts. In an emotional state, how we feel takes precedence over logic and fact. The good news is that we can change the old belief as soon as it is identified allowing us to make permanent changes to weight issues. The Food Voice Diet works on a deep level enhancing balance, feeling grounded and a sense of knowing that you are now on the right path. We need to do a little bit of weeding now and again with our food habits and beliefs to make sure our food voice is our friend not foe.

MOTIVATION TO CHANGE BELIEFS

A very successful method to help change old beliefs is to use the power of a future goal to keep you on track. Using a future event as a magnet to pull you forward is a great way to begin this diet. Once momentum kicks in, the release of uplifting energy gives you the extra boost you need to keep on track. Once you start to feel even a little bit better you are less likely to go back where you started.

FUTURE GOALS AND INTENTIONS

- Setting a weight loss goal.
- Losing weight to improve your health
- Changing your diet to boost energy levels.

- Wanting to be rid of constant food thoughts
- Going on holiday or a special event.
- Changing your diet to improve mental health and brain functionality.

HOW TO FORM NEW BELIEFS

1. "I have a really slow metabolism." NEW BELIEF: "I assumed I had a slow metabolism, but perhaps this was my weight excuse and now I can see that yo-yo dieting, eating the wrong food, eating too many carbs has caused my excess fat storage. My metabolism will work just fine if I make the right choices."

2. "I am big boned and have always been big which means I am doomed to stay that way." NEW BELIEF:
   "People said I was big boned as a youngster, but maybe this was just to make me feel better about being chubby. The label stuck and so did my weight. I may have a larger frame who knows, but I certainly do not have to accept the overweight part. My frame is nothing to do with being overweight and I now remove that old label which no longer applies to me. I am not that chubby child any longer and refuse to believe that I have to stay that way."

3. "All my family are overweight." NEW BELIEF: "I do not have to follow suit. We always had huge meals and snacked on all the wrong foods. I like eating, but this is making my life a misery. I can enjoy food I like on this diet and now I know which type of foods to limit I am going for it. I thought I was eating the right way by loading up on the pasta and bread and getting rid of

butter for a vegetable oil version. I thought I was always hungry because I had a big appetite. It all makes sense now I think about it."

4. "It is too difficult to diet, as I have to make separate meals for my family." **NEW BELIEF:** "A little bit more effort in meal planning and preparation, at least four nights a week, could really change how bad I am feeling about this weight gain. I can make the effort because I am worth it and I will be a happier mum once I get back in my old jeans again. My children can fit in with my new diet programme as most of the food is perfect for the children too and I can just eat less of the carbohydrate. I feel tired and lack energy, which is connected to what I have been eating. Wearing my old jeans is now my goal. This will motivate me to get started."

5. "I never have time for breakfast or lunch." **NEW BELIEF:** "I accepted this as part of my hectic schedule, so when I overeat in the evening I blame it on stress. I could prep a quick breakfast the night before and get organised to carry some snacks and lunch even if this was at least three out of my five working days. If that is what it will take to help me shift this weight I am doing it! I thought deep down that I was saving calories by missing meals, but now after reading this book I can see why that has not worked for me. I really believed missing meals would make me lose weight."

6. "I have a sweet tooth or I am a chocoholic." **NEW BELIEF:** "I do like chocolate of course who does not, but I know I eat more of it when I tell myself this. I have

such major cravings all day and I feel so out of balance and eat the chocolate just to feel OK for a while. I am so much larger now and I can see I need to change that belief because it really is not working. Of course, I will remain hooked on chocolate if I keep eating it because of what it is doing to my brain chemicals and that is why I have been eating even more of the stuff. At least I am not completely to blame, as I believed it was just part of me and I had to live with it."

7. "I cannot believe I can ever lose the weight and keep it off." NEW BELIEF: "After so many failed diets, I felt it was my entire fault as none of them worked. After reading this book I can see how my eating habits have caused my weight gain because I went too far, my diets were a punishment. There is light at the end of the tunnel. I am going to do it this time, as I now know exactly what I have been doing wrong. I am only going to eat the healthy foods I really enjoy."

8. "I am scared of letting go of certain foods I believe I need them to get through the day." NEW BELIEF: "I now know why eating less carbs works, plus I get to choose some yummy food treats I had always denied myself because I believed they were fattening. I like The Food Voice Diet food list, I have already decided on breakfast tomorrow, swapping food treats is a no brainer"

9. "My eating habits have been so bad for so long it is pointless trying to change." NEW BELIEF: "I have always had a bad diet, but where is the rule that states I am stuck with it. It is a bit of a challenge to make changes, but

what could be worse than how I feel now with this extra tummy. I can set new rules for myself and make a start it is only as difficult as I believe it to be. I believed I was destined to be fat. I can laugh now, but that is how I felt."

10. "I cannot resist eating the wrong foods." NEW BELIEF: "I have told myself that for so long because most of the time I felt so out of balance and went from one agitated state to the next with some junk food in between. I never felt well or even that full because of the cravings. I can see from reading this book what foods are addictive and why I have behaved this way. There is nothing wrong with me that a change of diet will not help. I now believe I can get balanced and in control with my craving and still enjoy delicious, healthy food."

11. "I just love eating, it is a hobby, also when I am tired I eat just as a pick me up." NEW BELIEF: "I can still be a foodie, but a different foodie. Just because I love food, does not mean I have to eat food that is draining my energy as this is ruining my life. I now choose to eat healthier food without chemical additives and processing. The Food Voice Diet food list gives me such a huge range of raw ingredients to create delicious meals. If I knew dieting tasted this good, I would have started years ago."

SOLUTIONS KEY 5 THE DIET PROGRAMME

The aim of The Food Voice Diet is to motivate you to change your current food voice to one that helps you choose the right foods for weight loss and to improve health and energy levels. The diet is based on real foods, which your body can convert to healthy tissues, providing you with energy, feeds your brain, helps you get rid of excess weight and tone up. Foods choices will focus on.

1. Protein

2. Fats

3. Carbohydrates

4. Vitamins, minerals and enzymes.

5. Real natural foods focusing on enjoyment, satisfaction, variety, health and weight loss. Mother nature has kindly provided us with such a wide range of delicious food on our planet. We are not designed to eat fake food as our bodies cannot process it.

This low carbohydrate diet offers a huge variety of meals and snacks, but the main aim is to reduce your carbohydrate intake. You can vary quantities to suit your needs and the speed at which you would like to lose weight. One of the main advantages of this diet is that the quantity of carbs can be varied to suit the following:

1. Your desired rate of weight loss

2. The amount of exercise and physical activity you engage in

3. You control the carbohydrates to fit in with your daily schedule

4. Fine-tune the amount of carbohydrate that is right for you to ensure you have plenty of energy during weight loss.

5. Choose one day a week (optional) to increase your daily allowance of carbohydrates without going overboard. This day off from low carbs is useful once you have reached your target weight or to provide you with a flexible day to fit in your social life.

WHAT ARE CARBOHYDRATES

The 2 types of carbs

1. Sugars such as sucrose, fructose and glucose are one type called simple carbohydrates. Examples include sugar, honey, jam, cakes, biscuits, milk chocolate, fruit juice, sodas, packaged breakfast cereals. This type should be limited or avoided.

2. Starch such as whole grain bread, rice, pasta and grains are the other and are called complex carbohydrates as they contain fibre. Fibre slows the absorption of sugar preventing blood sugar levels rising as fast. Vegetables, fruit, whole grains, beans, lentils, peas, oats, grains are complex carbs.

WHAT DO CARBS DO

Carbohydrates provide energy to be used throughout the body and brain; they are a quick release form of food able to reach the blood supply fast due to the speed of absorption. Some carbs provide nutrients and fibre to support and aid our health, but not in the sugar format as this food only provides empty calories which can cause many adverse reactions to our health and our ability to burn fat. Carbohydrates are beneficial but not essential to the diet in the same way as protein and dietary fat.

BENEFITS OF CARBOHYDRATES

1. An excellent provider of glucose for energy required by the body and brain

2. Provides energy for the body, allowing protein to carry out its job. Enough carbohydrate is required for your daily energy to prevent muscle being used for fuel. It is important not to reduce your carbs excessively for these reasons.

3. A good source of fibre from fruit and vegetables

4. To supply nutrients from complex carbohydrate foods

DISADVANTAGES OF EXCESS CARBOHYDRATE

1. High blood sugar and imbalances

2. High cholesterol and blood triglyceride levels.

3. Fatty liver. Over works the liver

4. Fat storage

5. Insulin and leptin resistance causing excessive fat
    storage and inability to control satiety and hunger
    signals.

6. Food addictions and eating issues, makes you more
    hungry, easy to overeat.

7. Lowered immunity. Robs you of Vitamin B, minerals
    and enzymes.

8. **Weight gain and lack of energy**

HOW DO CARBOHYDRATES AFFECT TRIGLYCERIDES (fat circulating in the bloodstream)

Carbohydrates contain virtually zero fat, which is why for
many years, the low fat diet was declared the healthiest diet
of all. Low fat and high carbohydrate dieting has not reduced
the problem of high cholesterol and blood triglycerides and
the related illnesses. A diet high in carbohydrate causes high
blood sugar stimulating insulin production. Insulin then
signals the liver to make fatty acids whereupon triglycerides
are produced and released into the bloodstream. Triglycerides
are produced from high carbohydrate diets and as the body
is unable to use all the food consumed is turns the carbs into
triglycerides to be stored as fat and some fat is left to float
freely around the bloodstream sticking to artery walls, which
can lead to heart disease. The worst combination of food to
consume is excess carbohydrates and dietary fat as you are
consuming two fat sources at once.

THE DANGER OF STORED FAT

Fat is stored in cells and is stored under the skin called subcutaneous fat, which is spread around the body. This fat is the type we focus on losing when we want to lose weight as it is stored on our hips, thighs, face, arms and back. The other fat stored around our middle and internal organs is called visceral fat. This fat holds the biggest health risk as it is active metabolically in a very toxic way as it excretes toxins to the bloodstream. Visceral fat contains more cortisol receptors and secretes molecules which increase inflammation. This has a knock on effect on other organs and even brain function. This fat pumps out substances called cykotines to the liver, which trigger the production of cholesterol and triglycerides resulting in your belly fat making you fatter outside of food consumption. Most people have no idea that visceral fat is negatively active and how important it is to lose weight and not just to look better in the mirror.

HEALTH RISKS of VISCERAL FAT

1. High blood pressure, triglycerides and cholesterol

2. Increased lipogenesis (fat creation).

3. Increased cortisol production. Cortisol helps baby fat cells grow (adipocytes)

4. Insulin and leptin resistance

5. Diabetes, certain cancers. Cancers feed on sugar.

6. Cardiovascular disease. Stroke from increased cholesterol and triglycerides.

7. Suppression of immune system

8. Memory and learning problems

9. Excess oestrogen metabolised by visceral fat

10. Feel good brain chemicals reduced. Alzheimer's disease, dementia

11. Places excess weight on our skeleton and joints,

12. Cortisol the stress hormone can actually cause a shift in subcutaneous fat to visceral fat because tummy fat is easier to access and utilize to meet the body's energy needs when we are stressed. Remember cortisol sends a message the body needs fuel to deal with stress. The more stressed, the more fuel is required. This is why stress causes hunger, then stores fat around the middle. In addition, our body is designed to store fat around the middle to keep our arms and legs free to allow movement and flexibility.

HOW CARBS MAKE US FAT

Carbohydrates turn to sugar promoting weight gain. In real terms, this food makes us "**eat more and want more**." Once sugar is consumed it lights a fire of desire in our brain which sends us messages, urging us to eat more without registering we are full. It confuses the normal appetite and fullness monitoring mechanism, which can leave us confused by our own behaviour. The sugar food voice is the worst voice of all, it can speak over you, interrupt, demand constant attention, turn you into a food obsessed sugar addict. The Food Voice Diet promotes fat burning and weight loss to help you to look and feel better. The emphasis is also strongly on health, especially the reduction of visceral fat which is detrimental to many medical issues.

REDUCE CARBOHYDRATES FOR WEIGHT LOSS

1. Reducing the overall consumption of carbs in meals, snacks and drinks.

2. Reducing the type of carbs you eat

3. Eating your carbohydrate allowance with fat and protein to avoid blood sugar spikes.

4. Aim to eat carbs with fibre to reduce the load on your blood sugar

5. Limit or exclude carbohydrate drinks such as soda and fruit juices as they cause insulin spikes.

6. Eat enough carbs for daily energy and preventing your body using muscle as a source of energy.

7. Ensure you consume coconut oil to supplement your energy levels (especially in the morning)

8. Eat enough carbs to ensure your body has enough energy to allow protein to do its job for your body.

9. Avoid sugar and processed food carbohydrates

10. Limit the amount of insulin released by limiting carbohydrates as, more insulin = more fat

11. High levels of insulin promote fat storage preventing fat loss

CARBOHYDRATE ALLOWANCE PER DAY

Weight Loss Level	Carbs Per Day
Fast Track Rapid weight loss	20-40 grams
Medium Level Steady weight loss	40-50 grams
Low Level Slow weight loss or maintenance	50-100 grams
Divide daily allowance between meals	

All levels depend on your daily level of activity. The more active you are the higher your carbohydrate requirements. (See back of book for food charts)

LIST OF FOOD WITH ONLY 15 GRAMS OF CARBOHYDRATE

- Slice of bread, half bagel, 6 inch tortilla, half pita bread

- 5 tablespoons of couscous

- Grains barley, 5 tablespoons

- 1 cup of milk, (cow, goat or sheep's)

- I apple

- 4 tablespoons pasta, rice or noodles

- I portion of berries

- 8 tablespoons of oatmeal

- 8 tablespoons squash

- 8 tablespoons black beans
- Quarter baked potato, 6 tablespoons boiled or mashed (or sweet potato)
- Yam 6 tablespoons
- Portion of soup average size
- Small serving of plain yogurt
- I corn on the cob
- Hummus 2 tablespoons
- 8 tablespoons of peas or sweet corn
- 3 tablespoons of flour or coconut flour (gluten and grain free)

Fat contains zero carbohydrate
Animal protein contains minimal levels of carbohydrate

VEGETABLES 5 GRAMS OF CARBOHYDRATE PER SERVING
(1 cup or 16 tablespoons)

Asparagus, artichoke, green beans, bean sprouts, broccoli, Brussel sprouts, cabbage, carrots, cauliflower, celery, cucumber, aubergine, leeks, mushrooms, onions, peppers,radishes, tomato, turnips, watercress, salad greens, spinach

WHAT IS PROTEIN

It is essential for health and survival

Proteins are large molecules made from amino acids. It is the second most abundant substance in the body, water being the first. Protein foods supply us with amino acids that are essential to our health and must be consumed daily, as it cannot be stored in the body. This category of food has many jobs and functions.

- A source of energy and a supply of nutrients

- To support healthy cell formation and functioning -Building and growth of muscle as muscle is made of protein. Protein supports muscle tone.

- For repair and maintenance, building of bones, muscles, cartilage, blood, hair, eyes, nails and skin.

- Immune and hormone health. Manufactures enzymes and functionality.

- Red blood cell production. Haemoglobin is a protein which carries oxygen.

- To assist the production of brain neurotransmitters such as dopamine.

TWO TYPES OF PROTEIN

Complete protein types contain more of the essential amino acids such as meat, fish, eggs and dairy products.
Incomplete protein types contain only some of the essential amino acids such as nuts, beans, grains and seeds. Ensure you have a good supply of complete proteins, but also to add variety to your diet by including incomplete proteins as they are also a good source of vitamins and minerals.

Eating too much protein can turn to glucose and be stored as fat. The daily protein allowance should be divided between your meals to be utilized properly as eating your daily allowance in one meal would be counterproductive. As this diet is a carbohydrate reduction regime it is essential to replace this void with healthy dietary fats. This diet will not work if you decide to cut out the fats and just eat protein with minimal carbohydrates. The section on fats will explain exactly what you will be depriving your body of by doing this and will be detrimental to your health. In addition, your mental health may be compromised, as the brain need healthy fats.

LACK OF PROTEIN

1. Muscle loss

2. Lowered immune system

3. Anaemia

4. Affected growth rates in children

5. Hypo-tension, low blood pressure

6. Healing and circulation affected

7. Weakening of the heart and respiratory system

ADVANTAGES OF PROTEIN FOR WEIGHT LOSS

Protein consumption does not cause an excess rise in blood sugar in the same way as carbohydrates which helps to limit the amount of insulin released. This provides a feeling of balance with regard to appetite control as protein is absorbed slowly and keeps blood sugar stable. The big plus protein holds for weight loss is that it keeps you full for longer than carbohydrates.

1. Improved appetite control

2. Feeling of satisfaction, satiety and fullness. Feel full longer.

3. Keeps the blood sugar stable, keeps you alert.

4. Helps relieve cravings and food addictions

5. Feeling balanced mentally and physically

6. Increases metabolism

7. Keeps muscle tone and muscle mass

8. Lowers blood pressure and helps reduce water retention

9. Provides the body with the necessary building and repair food

10. Protein is required to maintain and repair the heart muscle called the myocardial.

HOW MUCH PROTEIN IS REQUIRED EACH DAY

Approximately 0.8 to 1.5 grams of protein per kilo of body weight for adults, but teenagers require more for their growth. The average is approximately 50-90 grams of protein per day divided over the day. Large, tall people may require slightly more per meal. The ranges provided are to be used a guideline to ensure you to eat enough protein for health and weight loss, but not to excess. Fine tuning the diet is simple and after a week or two as you start to note which proteins work best for you in terms of keeping you full for longer, how much is too much and what is not enough, will become second nature to you. The guidelines listed below are approximate grams of protein in the average portion of meat and fish. If your chicken breast or meat portion is a little larger this is not what is classed as excessive consumption of protein, but to give you an idea of the portion size. If you are exercising on a regular basis you may need a little more protein than suggested.

PROTEIN CONTENT OF FOOD

Protein Food	Grams Protein
1 cup of milk (8 fl oz)	8
1 cup of raw milk can be substituted	8
3 oz or (more or less 1 chicken breast)	21
Chicken thigh on average	10
Chicken wing	6
3oz steak approx	28
Hamburger 4oz (meat only)	28
Pork chop average	22
3oz lamb or veal	30
3 oz ham	19
8 tablespoons cooked beans such as kidney (Contain more carbs than animal protein)	9
Nut butter 2 tbsp	8
8oz container of plain yogurt approx	11
2 egg omelette or scrambled	12
3 slices of bacon	9
3 oz sausage	18
3 oz piece of fish	21
Half cup cottage cheese	14
3 oz prawns	21
3 oz tuna	22
1 oz mozzarella brie, Camembert	6
Cheddar,	7-8
Parmesan	10

3oz converts to 85 grams in weight

EATING EXCESS PROTEIN

The Food Voice Diet promotes the consumption of complete proteins predominately, to ensure all the essential amino acids are consumed, but there are limits to the amount of protein as this is not a high protein diet. During the first two weeks on the diet, you may eat more protein than normal as you are adjusting to a new style of eating. If you engage in higher levels of exercise your protein requirements may increase.

• The body can only use a certain amount of protein in one day, any excess is stored as fat
• Excess protein metabolism strains the liver
• Digestion issues
• Fatigue, compromises energy levels
• Lack of calcium as excess protein utilizes extra calcium
• Can affect blood sugar and insulin release in excess. However, it is difficult to over consume to the same extent as carbohydrates.

THE ROLE DIETARY FATS

They are essential for health and survival

It is fair to say that the subject of which type of fat to eat is a complicated topic. Many dieters have become ultra concerned about consuming fat and have tried to avoid it in the hope of losing weight. We ponder as to whether we should eat a low fat diet? Or is saturated fat the enemy? What is trans fat? Does eating fat make me fat? This book will provide information on the role of each type of fat and why you should include it in your diet. You will learn why not to skip on consuming fat and which types of fat to avoid and why. I will explain the type of fats present in the food and show you why certain foods you may have been advised not to eat actually contain a variety of fats, not only saturated fat. Take beef for example which is normally classed as a supply of saturated fat without mentioning that beef also contains omega 3 fats (especially grass fed beef), conjugated linoleic acid(CLA) a fat which helps fight high blood pressure, osteoporosis, and certain cancers. Do not be frightened of eating healthy fat in moderation, as it will help you to lose weight if you combine it with the correct carbohydrate reduction. **Eating fat has no effect on blood sugar therefore there is no insulin response to healthy fat consumption.**

The fat we eat comes in four categories called saturated, polyunsaturated, monounsaturated and trans fats and in each category, there are many types of fat. The body can process all the fats apart from trans fats, which act as a toxin to the system.

Saturated fat. Animal protein, dairy products. Non animal sources such as coconut and palm oil. These fats are solid and do not normally go rancid even when cooking at high temperatures.

Monounsaturated fat (unsaturated fat) Olive oil, olives, cashew nuts, almonds, hazelnuts, avocados. Omega 6. Linoeic acid is an omega 6 fatty acid. Sources include leafy vegetables, seeds and walnuts. These fats tend to be liquid at room temperature and are not stable when cooking at high temperatures.

Polyunsaturated fat. Essential fatty acids (unsaturated fat) Omega 3. Linolenic acid is an omega 3 fatty acid. Sources include salmon, tuna, sardines, shellfish, omega 3 eggs, flaxseed oil and grass fed beef. This fat, in the form of oil, can go rancid very quickly and must never be used for cooking. It is important to eat enough of the essential omega 3 and 6 fatty acids in balance as many people have an excess of 6, but not enough 3 which can result in inflammation, high blood pressure, blood clots, lack of immunity, depression, cancer, digestive disorders and weight gain.

Processed polyunsaturated oils such as corn, soy-bean, sunflower and safflower are not recommended. These oils are not in their natural state and are hard to process in the liver. Manufacturers use genetically modified crops to maximise profits, the crops are heavily treated with pesticides and then heavily processed to be able to extract oil from the seeds. These oils can easily become rancid when heat is applied and by exposure to oxygen. Free radicals are released from these unstable fats, which are invisible to the human eye, but cause damage to cell membranes, red blood cells, skin tissue, organs and can cause premature ageing. Free radicals can also damage blood vessels and cause a build up of arterial plaque and immune system dysfunction, increase uric acid formation and mental decline.

Trans fat (processed saturated fat) is manufactured liquid vegetable oil made solid using high heat and adding hydrogen. These fats are hard to metabolise by the liver as unsaturated fat is chemically altered to become a saturated fat that adds shelf life and gives it a different texture, which makes this cheap fat very popular in food manufacturing. This type of fat can raise the bad cholesterol levels (LDL), lower good cholesterol (HDL) and affect heart health. This product is toxic to the liver.

Sources. Margarine and spreads, shortening, cake mixes, ice cream, non dairy creamers, microwave popcorn, milk shakes, salad dressings, ready meals, fried fast food, processed cakes and biscuits, junk food products, pies, pizzas, chips and fries. Low fat processed food can contain trans fat.

THE HEALTH BENEFITS TO EATING GOOD FATS

1. Fats taste good and make you feel full. (It is difficult to overeat fat on its own, but mixed with sugar and other carbohydrates such as chocolate, cake or crisps. It is easy to overeat these products and become food addicted.)

2. Fat is needed to transport fat-soluble vitamins such as A, D, E and K. and to absorb minerals such as calcium. There is no point ensuring you consume these vitamins but do not eat enough fat to utilize them.

3. Provides energy for the body. The heart prefers to use fat as its primary fuel source.

4. Fat provides essential fatty acids that the body cannot make itself.

5. The formation and maintenance of cells, plus the function of the cells as receptors of messages, which

can affect the ability of the body to burn fat stores. You need to eat good fat to burn fat.

6. Healthy bones, eyes, hair, skin and teeth

7. Good brain function and improved mental health. The feel good factor is so important for weight loss success.

8. Lowers inflammation. Improved immunity.

9. Cushions the body and helps to protect the skeleton

10. Childhood growth and brain development

11. Good hormone production

12. Blood clotting

13. Lowers the risk of osteoporosis.

14. Certain fats help lower cholesterol

15. Helps promote better moods by improving nutritional health

SATURATED FAT BENEFITS

Saturated fats are natural, good for our health and essential to the functions of the body. Trans fat is the only saturated fat that should be avoided as it is a processed fat. Saturated fats contain a mixture of monounsaturated and polyunsaturated fat, the same also applies to animal protein foods.

1. The lung airspaces have a coating made up of entirely saturated fatty acids. If no saturated fat is made available other fat substitutes are made which can cause lung and breathing problems.

2. Saturated fats helps the absorption of calcium

3. Brain function depends on saturated fat to repair and maintain itself as the brain is made in part of saturated fat.

4. Saturated fat helps the cells send signals and messages such as releasing the correct levels of insulin.

5. Unhealthy cells, lacking in saturated fat are the cause of a lowered immune system.

6. Saturated fat is needed to transport the essential fats omega 3 and 6 and to ensure the fats can be utilized correctly in the tissues.

7. The fat around the heart is made up of saturated fat, the body can draw on this fat when it is under stress. The heart uses saturated fat as the preferred source of energy.

8. Without enough saturated fats in our cell walls, polyunsaturated fat is used as a substitute causing cell weakness.

HEALTHY NATURAL SATURATED FATS

1. Organic coconut oil (resistant to rancidity)

2. Palm oil

3. Organic beef tallow (beef fat)

4. Butter especially from grass fed cows. Organic ghee (clarified butter)

5. Free range lard (pork fat)

6. Free range goose and duck fat

7. Dairy products

8. Meat and fish

9. Nuts and nut oil

The less our food is processed in anyway including low fat versions of real food the easier the body can metabolize and use this food for maximum health. Manufactured, processed oils using high temperatures and chemicals to extract the oil from grains cannot compete with natural oils from real food. The saturated fat to avoid is trans fat, which is an imitation saturated fat, devised by manufacturers to cut production costs. The trans fat concept was great for business, but bad for our health. The Food Voice Diet aids weight loss whilst at the same time promoting brain nutrition, which means consuming healthy fats. Mental balance is essential to successful long-term weight loss along with ensuring your energy levels help support your lifestyle to get the maximum pleasure out of each day.

COCONUT OIL AND WEIGHT LOSS

The Food Voice Diet recommends the use of coconut oil as the main choice of fat for energy as it stimulates metabolism due to the structure of the fat called medium chained triglycerides (MCT's.). This oil can be metabolised for a quick source of energy. The digestion of coconut oil differs from other dietary fats, it does not utilise bile or enzymes from the pancreas. The liver is able to process this oil quickly and easily giving you a wonderful surge of energy. Coconut oil does not cause blood sugar issues and insulin spikes which helps keep your appetite and satiety under control. This oil has anti fungal, anti viral, anti parasitic and antimicrobial properties.

BENEFITS OF ORGANIC COCONUT OIL

- Increases metabolism assisting weight loss
- Promotes a healthy heart
- Increases and improves energy levels
- Improves thyroid function
- Improves skin
- Resistance to viruses and bacteria.
- Aids digestion. Helps reduce inflammation and leaky gut.
- Zero insulin release, an alternative source of energy for people with insulin resistance who struggle to obtain energy from glucose (carbohydrates)
- Aids mineral and nutrient absorption especially vitamins B, A, D, E, K and certain proteins.
- Helps lower (LDL) bad cholesterol and improves good cholesterol (HDL)
- Normalize blood clotting
- Does not circulate in the blood stream like other fats, avoiding build up in fat cells and arteries.
- Helps satiety and appetite control
- Does not affect blood sugar
- Can improve brain function and cognitive performance
- Feeling grounded

MONOUNSATURATED FAT

Such as olive oil is beneficial to our health. It is not recommended to use these oils for high temperature cooking. One of the main benefits most people are already aware of is lowering the risk of heart disease by:

1. Lowering the bad cholesterol LDL whilst maintaining the good cholesterol HDL

2. Normalize blood clotting

BENEFITS OF MONOUNSATURATED FATS

1. Stabilizing blood sugar response

2. Antioxidants protecting the body from inflammation

HEALTHY SOURCES

1. Olive oil, olives. Good quality olive oil is pressed without the use of chemical solvents and high temperatures as used in the production of sunflower and safflower oils.

2. Avocados and oil

3. Nut butters

4. Macadamia nut oil

5. Sesame oil

6. Pumpkin seeds

POLYUNSATURATED FATS

Essential fatty acids must be added to your diet in a balanced way as most people have a high omega 6 and a low omega 3 ratio. Cooking with high heat can strip this oil of fatty acids.

OMEGA 3 BENEFITS

1. Helps organs function properly

2. Cell activity and cell wall formation

3. Oxygen circulation

4. Red blood cell function

5. Blood clot prevention

6. Prevents loss of memory

7. Eyes, nails and hair

8. Regulates heartbeat

9. Immune system support

10. Mental health and brain function

11. Regulates blood pressure

12. Reduces inflammation

13. Improves insulin response

14. Concentration

Sources. Walnuts, sesame and sunflower seeds, salmon, sardines, shrimp, scallops, tuna, spinach, grass fed beef, grass fed butter and cod liver oil.

OMEGA 6 BENEFITS

1. Healthy skin

2. Fights cancer cells

3. Helps arthritis

4. Brain function, growth and development

5. Allergy prevention

6. Muscle development

7. Nervous system function

8. Improves mood and energy

Sources. Pistachios, pecans, olive oil, chicken, egg yolks, grain fed meat, peanut butter, flaxseed oil, bacon fat. Most people have adequate levels of good omega 6 intake, but due to the consumption of high levels of sugar and trans fats the benefits are reduced. It is important not to cook with omega 6 oils as they are not heat stable and are prone to oxidation and can turn your good cholesterol (HDL) into the bad cholesterol (LDL) the main culprit of clogged arteries.

DANGERS OF EATING TOO MUCH OMEGA 6 VERSUS OMEGA 3

It is important to consume enough omega 3 to balance the intake of omega 6, as it is easy to find foods with an abundance of 6 and miss the very important omega 3. By reducing foods cooked in polyunsaturated vegetable oils and increasing foods with omega 3 it is easy to not only get this ratio balanced, but also reduce the damage to health caused by rancid vegetable oils.

The 6 to 3 imbalance is associated with many inflammatory diseases such as

1. Arthritis

2. Cancer

3. Insulin and leptin resistance

4. Obesity

5. Irritable bowel syndrome

6. Asthma

7. Immune issues

8. Mental health issues

9. Type 2 diabetes

10. Coronary artery disease

11. Osteoporosis

IDEAL FATS FOR COOKING

Dietary fats are a mixture of three types of fat. People generally assume that lard for example is completely saturated fat or that olive oil is best for cooking.

1. Coconut oil. Saturated, monounsaturated and polyunsaturated, fat, vitamins E, K, choline iron

2. Palm oil. Saturated, monounsaturated and polyunsaturated fat vitamins E, K, choline
3. Organic Ghee. Saturated monounsaturated and polyunsaturated fat, omega 3 and 6, vitamin A, E, K, calcium, magnesium, phosphorus, potassium, sodium, zinc and selenium, conjugated linoliec acid.(CLA)
4. Grass fed butter. Saturated, monounsaturated, polyunsaturated, vitamins A, D, E, K, manganese, chromium, zinc, copper, selenium, iodine, omega 3 and 6, CLA
5. Organic lard. Saturated, monounsaturated and polyunsaturated fat, selenium, zinc, choline, vitamin E
6. Goose fat. Saturated, monounsaturated and polyunsaturated omega 3 and 6, selenium, vitamin E
7. Duck fat. Saturated, monounsaturated and polyunsaturated fat, vitamin E, choline, selenium
8. Olive oil mono-unsaturated, saturated and polyunsaturated, vitamin E, selenium, zinc.(Low temperature cooking only)

OILS FOR DRESSING or to DRIZZLE

1. Olive oil. Saturated, monounsaturated and polyunsaturated, omega 3 and 6, vitamin E, K, betaine, calcium, iron, potassium, sodium
2. Sesame oil. Polyunsaturated, monounsaturated and saturated, omega 3 and 6, vitamin E, K, choline
3. Avocado oil. Monounsaturated, polyunsaturated and saturated

4. Flaxseed oil. Polyunsaturated, monounsaturated and saturated, vitamin E, choline
5. An oil mix made of coconut oil, olive oil and sesame oil or other variations. Store in the fridge.

COMPOSITION OF DIETARY FATS			
Fat	Saturated	Mono	Poly
Olive Oil	14	77	9
Chicken Fat	31	47	22
Lard	41	47	12
Beef Fat	52	44	4
Palm Oil	51	39	10
Butter	66	30	4
Coconut Oil (MCT)	92	6	2

DAILY ADDITIONAL FAT ALLOWANCE

Coconut oil is the number one choice of dietary fat in The Food Voice Diet as it provides an ideal source of energy plus many other health benefits. The energy derived from coconut oil is experienced as pure effortless vitality as opposed to the wired energy obtained from sugar and caffeine. The oil is not digested in the same way as other fats, it is much lighter on your digestive system. Consuming coconut oil on a daily basis enhances mental well being and feeling grounded.

Breakfast up to 1 tablespoon of coconut oil is the preferred fat for weight loss and boosting energy levels. Butter and other fats can be substituted accordingly, but if cooking do

not use unsaturated or polyunsaturated fats. Example 1 tsp for coffee, 1 tsp for toast and 1 tsp to cook eggs
Lunch and snacks up to 2 tablespoons divided between cooking method, bulletproof drink and any fresh cream or mayonnaise. Example 2 tsp to cook lunch, 5 tsp cream for berries, 1 tsp bulletproof tea.

Evening meals up to 2 tablespoons as above. 3 tsp to cook meal, 1 tsp butter for veg, I cup of cocoa hot milk with 1 tsp of coconut oil.

The daily allowance depends on your height frame and activity level. If you are experiencing undue tiredness as you reduce your carbohydrate intake this is a sign your fat intake may not be high enough for your energy needs.
The concept is to exchange the energy from carbohydrates and replace with dietary fat, which does not cause insulin spikes and fat storage if consumed in moderation. I teaspoon of fat is approximate 40 calories.
I tablespoon = 3 teaspoons

CONCLUSION

Excess carbohydrate causes fat storage and insulin related problems despite being a good source of quick energy for the body and brain. By reducing carbohydrates for energy and using healthy fats for energy, the body avoids insulin and fat storage problems and is able to focus on fat burning. Healthy fats do not cause weight gain if used in moderation and in combination with this low carbohydrate diet. Fat, does not raise insulin levels. Less insulin = less stored fat. Fats and protein are highly beneficial and essential to the body in comparison to carbohydrates, which can be reduced and replaced. Fat has zero effect on insulin levels. One of the huge pluses in exchanging healthy fats for carbohydrate for energy is satiety. A higher fat, lower carb meal with adequate protein provides a much higher level of satisfaction and fullness not only after consumption, but also for many hours afterwards. The satisfaction level blunts not only the appetite, but the desire for sweet and starchy foods is drastically reduced. High carbohydrate, low fat meals increase the desire for more carbohydrates despite being full after eating. It is common to crave more carbohydrate such as chocolate, sugar desserts and biscuits after this type of meal due to blood sugar and insulin level fluctuations resulting in an out of control food voice.

BREAKFAST LUNCH AND DINNER

The Food Voice Diet focus is on healthy low carbohydrate foods, healthy fats and adequate levels of protein, to keep you and your brain happy and satisfied. Breakfast is very important for the obvious reason of providing fuel and energy for the day, but also this meal should really start you off on a good note mentally. A good start at breakfast sets the theme for the remainder of the day, keeping eating in balance. Breakfast should definitely include the type of food you like so much it is worth getting out of bed for. You need to fuel up, but why not get to feel good for the next 3 to 4 hours whilst feeling a boost from your good brain chemicals. Making healthy feel good choices feels great. The alternative is to eat something you regret which affects your blood sugar, leaves you feeling guilty whilst you ride the hunger imbalance roller coaster. A good breakfast does not need to be time consuming if you are in a rush to get to work. You are not counting calories, but you do have to limit your carbohydrate and ensure you add protein and fat to carbs you do eat. There are people who never eat breakfast and in this case you can drink your breakfast by adding coconut oil to coffee with full fat milk and a few nuts and you are good to go.

SUGGESTIONS BREAKFAST MENU

Aim for protein, nutrients, healthy fats, limited carbohydrates.
Include food you really enjoy eating.

- I slice of toast with grass fed butter and cheese - optional Marmite to taste
- I milky coffee with full fat milk add 1-3 tsp of organic coconut oil. 1- 4 walnuts
- I cup of warm milk, 1-3 tsp of coconut milk, 2 walnuts or 2 Brazil nuts
- Omelette with tuna and tomato or any other protein and vegetable
- Bacon and eggs (nitrate free bacon is best)
- Cheese and nuts with tomato or celery
- Mozzarella with avocado drizzle with olive oil
- Mozzarella or Camembert with bacon
- Eggs 2-3 cooked in grass fed butter, mushrooms optional
- Sausage (nitrate free) and tomato cooked in coconut oil.
- Scrambled eggs with smoked salmon, raw spinach and chopped parsley on top.

- Porridge oats with 1 tsp grass fed butter or coconut oil add up to 1 tbsp of fresh cream (soak oats in water overnight to improve digestion) berries, cinnamon, crushed flax seeds or nutmeg optional
- Berries with full fat plain or Greek yogurt. Organic frozen berries can be used.
- Pancakes made with coconut flour with sausage or bacon.
- Gammon and tomatoes topped with fresh parmesan shavings.
- Eggs Benedict
- Fish roe on grass fed buttered toast.
- Organic nut butter on slice of toast with bacon topping.
- Mushrooms, egg, sausage or bacon

BULLET PROOF COFFEE OR TEA

Coconut oil can be added to tea and coffee between 1 tsp to 1 tablespoon or make a 50-50 blend with grass fed butter. I tablespoon equals 3 teaspoons. 1 square of 99% dark chocolate can be added instead of butter. Coconut oil and dark chocolate make a great combination. Keep the chocolate in the freezer once opened to avoid the fat content going rancid. This beverage will not impact on your insulin levels, it provides a wonderful source of energy and it certainly has the 'Feel amazing' factor. 1 cube of chocolate = 1 tsp of your fat content for breakfast.

Avoid processed breakfast cereals, they contain preservatives, high levels of carbohydrates, genetically modified soy, high fructose corn syrup, chemicals, colours, flavourings, sodium and trans fat.

HOW MUCH SHOULD I EAT

Specific portions have not been included in the breakfast list, as the amount of protein a short narrow framed woman may eat will vary compared to a 6-foot large framed male. THE AIM is to eat enough to meet your protein requirements plus having enough energy until lunchtime, BUT do not eat to excess to ensure you lose weight. Finding the optimal level for breakfast, lunch and dinner will soon become second nature to you. (Refer to protein and carb charts at the back of the book)

TEA AND COFFEE

Tea and coffee can be consumed with meals to avoid the negative effects of caffeine on an empty stomach otherwise still or sparkling water can be substituted with food. Try and avoid drinking caffeine outside of mealtimes and stick to simple water to maintain your energy and keep your body working efficiently.

LUNCH MENU

Lunch can often be another meal which is rushed, but fuelling up is essential to make sure you keep your blood sugar stable and replenish your energy stores. It is easy to be so busy and skip lunch or to delay it until you get over hungry. Remember your brain is using 20% of your food intake for fuel, give your brain a chance to recover from the morning's work by re-fuelling. You will feel and work better after eating lunch plus your metabolism needs to keep active or it may slow down thinking a famine is on the way.

Yet again, you need to focus on enjoying your lunch and feel satisfied. Getting out of the sandwich habit will help to reduce the amount of carbs you eat on a daily basis. Bread can be one of the most difficult food habits to change if you are used to relying on bread for breakfast and lunch as easy options. One slice of bread is 15 grams of carbohydrate, which can easily use up your daily allowance and slow down your weight loss if you are eating 3 or 4 slices per day. You do not have to give up bread, but simply cut down. Open sandwiches with more protein than bread help to solve this problem or alternative bread days, one on and one off, until you find you are enjoying other food combinations as bread become less of an issue.

LUNCH TIPS

1. Open sandwiches with extra protein filling. Drizzle with your favourite oil or use delicious grass fed butter giving you a rich supply of vitamins D, A, E and K. This butter also contains manganese, zinc, copper, selenium, chromium iodine, omega 3 and 6 fatty acids and conjugated linoleic acid.
2. Serve sandwiches with a salad or top with a tomato, celery or avocado or any other vegetable.
3. Take lunch to work with you. Keep a supply of coconut oil at work to add to your coffee or tea. Use left-over meat or fish from the night before. Hot soup or casseroles can be heated up in a thermal pot and taken to work if you prefer a hot meal.

4. Vary your lunches as much as possible to ensure a wide range of food is eaten plus you receive a cross section of vitamins and minerals.
5. Keeping your carbohydrate levels balanced keeps excess hunger and cravings under control for the rest of the afternoon.
6. Roast chicken take away with a salad
7. Kebab with vegetables
8. Tandoori chicken with salad
9. Chinese chicken stir-fry with vegetables or Thai coconut curry with vegetables.
10. Many supermarkets sell hot food such as roast chicken and other meats and salads, which are a good alternative to fast fried foods.
11. All day breakfast avoiding fried items.

Wash all fruits and vegetables thoroughly to remove toxins from fertilizers and pesticides

EXAMPLE MIX AND MATCH 7 DAY SIMPLE 15 minute MENUS

Choose the complex carbohydrates you prefer to accompany your meals, vary quantities accordingly

Day	Pick your breakfast	Choose lunch	Decide on dinner
1	Greek yogurt, blueberries, 1-2 chopped walnuts	Tandoori chicken, half nan bread, salad	Steak with pepper cream sauce 3 veg, 3 tbsp sweet potato.
2	Bacon, eggs mushrooms	Open grilled tuna sandwich topped with cheese, spinach	Grilled pork, 1 tbsp pasta, cream cheese, chives. 3 veg.
3	Porridge oats, 1 tsp coconut oil, 1 tsp fresh cream, cinnamon	All day breakfast not fried	Baked salmon with garlic butter, pesto, 3 veg. 2 tbsp couscous
4	Scrambled egg, smoked salmon, avocado	Home made beef broth, berries and 1 tbsp cream	Tuna steak, tomato, garlic, salsa, 2 veg. Dark chocolate 2 squares
5	Gammon, tomato or half bagel, cream cheese and smoked salmon	Meat or fish kebab with roasted vegetables, half pitta bread	Chicken coconut curry, corn on cob, brown rice.
6	Coconut pancake, sausage or bacon (substitute coconut flour in pancake recipe)	Lamb chop, 2 tbsp rice 2 buttered vegetables	Prawn, fish or meat stir fry, avocado Glass of red wine
7	Cheese on toast with marmite or egg and bacon.	2 tbsp hummus, with mozzarella or brie and celery	Sunday roast with 3 veg. 1 potato, 1 Yorkshire pudding, gravy, I glass red wine. Berries and cream, dark chocolate 1 square.

ADDITIONS

Bullet proof tea or coffee up to 3 per day, cod liver oil supplement, barley grass drink 2 per day. Fruit, bread and other higher carbs foods can be limited for the fast track version of The Food Voice Diet. Minerals and vitamins are supplemented by the barley grass drink. Use coconut oil wherever possible for cooking. Drink 10 glasses of water per day. A slow cooker is ideal for soups, curries and casseroles. Choose one day a week (optional) to increase your daily allowance of carbohydrates without going overboard. This day off from low carbs is useful once you have reached your target weight or to provide you with a flexible day to fit into your social life

SNACKS

After you have adjusted to eating less carbohydrates your appetite will stabilize and find a normal rhythm. If you are eating correctly on The Food Voice Diet, you will not find snacks necessary as your body will be using stored fat for energy in between meals. During the initial phase of the diet, snacking can be useful whilst adjusting. If you find the need for snacks, you will need to establish if you are eating enough protein and healthy fats for your body type and energy needs. Check if you are following the carbohydrate rules and not eating too many carbs in one meal causing an increase in appetite. If you need to snack due to a delay in mealtimes, or you have not eaten enough during your previous meals or experiencing an energy drain, the following can be used as guidelines.

- Do not eat carbohydrates without protein (especially fruit)
- Be prepared with nuts and seeds in your bag or at work. Nuts are an ideal snack as long as you do not eat huge quantities.
- Small amounts of cheese and celery
- Tuna or smoked or tinned salmon
- Hard-boiled egg
- Slice of ham and tomato
- Berries and plain or Greek yogurt
- Small portion of home- made soup
- 1 tsp of coconut oil and herbal or fresh ginger tea with a few macadamia nuts.
- **Organic barley grass powder** (Best choice for weight loss)

Try a very small snack first as you may well find that on this diet you do not need the volume of snacks you once ate on a higher carbohydrate diet. The ideal snack for weight loss is barley grass. Many people are surprised how a little snack now satisfies their hunger. Check also that your hunger sign is not a call for water as the two signals feel the same and can be easily confused. If your sudden hunger is a result of stress, find another way to reduce the stress instead of starting to eat. Drink some water, take a deep breath and work on a solution to the stress as opposed to using food.

DINNER GUIDELINES

Ideally, dinner is the time of the day you get to take a little more time to enjoy your meal, but if you are rushing out there are still many great tasty options to choose from according to your palate and budget. Leftovers and cooking extra for the freezer can help to cut a few corners.

1. Choose meals, herbs and spices you love to eat. Look forward to your meals and savour every mouthful.
2. Any meat or fish cooked with healthy cooking oil. Vegetables or salad. Coconut cream or fresh cream can be added to sauces. All cuts of meats, including organ meats such as liver. Game is also a good source of protein. Meat can be lightly trimmed and the skin of poultry included.
3. Grass fed butter or other oils of choice 1 tsp can be added to any cooked vegetables
4. Olive oil or real mayonnaise for salad. Other oils can be added from the polyunsaturated list for dressing and drizzle
5. Tinned tomato, or puree can be used for any sauces.
6. Slow cookers are very useful for cheaper cuts of meat and for busy people who tend to use takeaways and ready meals
7. Use organic fresh or dried herbs
8. Cook by any method apart from deep fat frying
9. Control the carbohydrate content of your meal by checking on the chart to see which vegetables and fruits are low carbohydrate depending on how much weight you want to lose

10. The amount of sugar in carbohydrates is released slowly when consumed with protein and fat. High carbohydrate vegetables such as corn and carrots served with butter and eaten with a meal will not affect the blood sugar as much.

11. All meals can be consumed with potatoes, pasta, rice, bread or the carbohydrate of your choice, but in small portions. This way you will not feel deprived of your favourite meals or look as though you are on a major diet when you are eating with other people.

12. Add omega 3 oils after meals are cooked on high heat to avoid destroying the benefits of the oil.

13. Mix oils together for a salad dressing or a dressing for meat and fish, i.e. Coconut, olive and walnut.

14. Organic frozen vegetables can help save time and preparation.

15. Fermented vegetables and products are beneficial to help balance good bacteria in the gut, also aids mineral absorption

16. Cook extra and freeze for lazy days.

17. Keep a list of the meals you really enjoyed. It is easy to forget when it comes to meal planning.

18. High fibre vegetables, approximately 3-4 portions per day.

19. Unrefined salt adds essential minerals, unlike processed table salt which undermines health.

20. Fresh lemon or lime juice added to cooked meat or fish as a dressing alongside olive oil to help boost vitamin C levels.

21. Variety is important, meals should include a selection of healthy fats plus vary your choice of proteins and

vegetables. You may not be cooking with olive oil, it can be drizzled over cooked meat or fish.

22. Broths and soups made from meat or fish bones. Ideal for slow cookers. Miso soup is a fermented product, additional protein and fat consumption will be required to make a balanced meal.

23. Avoid MSG. Monosodium glutamate is a man made additive. It is a savoury flavour enhancer helping cheap ingredients taste good. It can cause headaches, sweating, confusion and lack of concentration. It is contained in many processed foods such as crisps, crackers, ready meals, and soups and can trigger excessive appetite. It is hidden under the names hydrolysed vegetable protein, textured vegetable protein, hydrolysed yeast extract, textured whey or soy protein and plant protein extract.

24. Temperature. Try to avoid eating food straight from the fridge as taste and flavour improves at room temperature. Food is hard to chew when it is too hot which can cause digestive problems. Digestion begins in the mouth, make the most of the delicious food you have chosen and really enjoy the taste as long as possible. Take your time to eat and savour every mouthful.

DESSERTS

Fresh or frozen fruit with fresh cream is the optimal dessert providing nutrients, variety and taste. Fruit should not be eaten in between meals as it raises blood sugar. Dried fruit is very high in sugar and best avoided until you reach your target weight. Fruit can be served with a coconut pancake cooked in coconut oil. Greek or plain yogurt with optional chopped nuts, berries, cinnamon or nutmeg. Small amounts of dark chocolate 70% and over once or twice per week if required. It is a good source of iron, copper and magnesium, antioxidants and flavanols. 1 oz of dark chocolate is 15-16 grams of carbs. 1 square = 3.2 grams. Lindt 99% has zero grams of sugar. All desserts must be included in your carb content for the whole meal. Some people prefer to eat less carbohydrate with their main course and save a healthy carbohydrate for dessert on certain days or weekends. The Food Voice Diet gives you flexibility to make the choices, as you may prefer to eat berries and cream one day instead of potato and pasta with your main meal as your carb allowance.

DRINKS

Processed shop bought fruit juices have very high levels of sugar especially fructose, the processing takes most of the fibre and the skin from fruit causing insulin spikes. The same applies to home juiced fruit drinks as most of the fibre is removed making the sugar release rapidly into the bloodstream. Juices made from whole fruit where the fibre and skin are included are preferable, but drink in moderation to avoid insulin spikes.

- Water at least 10 glasses a day. Keep water at your workstation or close by you as a reminder as it is easy to forget to drink water regularly. The process of burning stored fat requires water to carry out this task efficiently.

- Smoothies made with whole milk and berries and/or coconut milk. (Include in carb allowance)
- Tea, coffee, green tea, 3 per day maximum as they contain caffeine
- Barley grass in between meals, which also doubles up as a snack.
- Ginger tea with crushed fresh ginger, fresh lemon and lime with, Coconut oil is optional. Caffeine free herbal teas without artificial flavours.
- Hot milk and 2 tsp organic cocoa (approx 10 grams of carbs) or hot milk with 1 tsp of coconut oil, 1 square of dark chocolate
    (Note all drinks with milk and chocolate constitute part of carb allowance)

SUPPLEMENTS

Cod liver oil supplies omega 3 plus vitamins A and D. Half to one teaspoon daily is recommended, preferably in the morning. Carlson's is an excellent brand which can be ordered on line from Amazon.

BENEFITS OF COD LIVER OIL

- Ideal for people who do not eat oily fish or not on a regular basis.
- Good cod liver oil supplies a good ratio of vitamins A and D (do not take if pregnant)
- Vitamin A supports eyesight and skin and helps the body absorb iron. Vitamin D for bone health and immunity.

- Provides both EPA and DHA - types of omega 3. ALA omega 3 is found in plants and seeds are not as beneficial as EPA and DHA.
- Arthritis relief, healthy joints
- Aids muscle pain
- Heart functionality, reduces blood triglycerides
- Fights inflammation, promotes wound healing
- Blood vessel elasticity, lowering blood pressure
- Helps brain and mental health
- Psoriasis relief
- Soothes asthma
- Protects against bone loss
- Healthy digestive tract

BENEFITS OF BARLEY GRASS
This is sprouted from barley seeds and harvested when the leaves are young where enzymes and nutrients are abundant. This product unlike certain vitamin pills does not contain synthetic vitamins which can be labelled "natural" even if they are made in a laboratory.

BARLEY GRASS POWDER
Mix 1 to 2 teaspoons per day into a glass of cold or room temperature mineral water. Ideally consumed two to three hours after a meal for maximum benefit, drink immediately after mixing. Green Magma is an excellent product available from Amazon. It is handy to carry around as a snack and easily mixed into a small bottle of mineral water.

BARLEY GRASS NUTRITION
Vitamins. A and B's 1, 2, 3, 6, 12, vitamins C, E, F K, folic acid, choline, niacin, panthothenic acid

Minerals: Calcium, zinc, sodium, selenium, potassium, phosphorus, nickel, magnesium, boron chloride. Chromium, cobalt, copper, iodine, iron, silicon, sulphur.
Antioxidants. Alpha carotene, beta carotene, chlorophyll, superoxide dismutase, catalase,
Amino acids. Alanine, arginine, aspartic acid, choline, cystine, glutamic acid, glycine malic, histidine nitrate, isoleucine, lysine, methionine, phenylalanine, proline, serine, threonine, tryptophan, tyrosine, valine
Enzymes. Aspartate aminotransferase, catalase, cytochrome oxidase, DNase, fatty acid oxidase, hexokinase, dehydrogenase, reductase, peroxidise, phospholipase, polyphenoloxidase, RNase, superoxide dismutase, transyhydrogenase.

- Contains 30 times more vitamin B1 and 11 times the amount of calcium in cow's milk. (Cod liver oil helps calcium absorption) It has 6.5 times as much carotene and almost 5 times the iron content of spinach, 6 times vitamin C than oranges .
- Contains organic sodium which helps dissolve calcium deposits in the joints
- Aids digestion and production of hydrochloric acid in the stomach.
- Contains superoxide dismutase a powerful antioxidant
- It is 45% protein made of 18 amino acids including 8 essentials the body cannot make.
- Keeps the acid alkaline balance for optimum health
- Enzyme content is high, up to 1, 000 varieties. (The spark plugs for body processes)
- Propionic acid, an enzyme that helps lower blood cholesterol.

- Aids blood circulation and formation of haemoglobin and red blood cells. Helps lower blood pressure
- Helps stabilize blood sugar
- Helps remove toxins, improves skin and complexion.
- Contains chlorophyll helping to purify the liver, is anti-bacterial, rejuvenates and rebuilds bodily tissues.
- Is an excellent source of fibre.
- Aids stress management
- If you are cutting down on fruit consumption to reduce sugar intake this is an essential supplement providing a supply of fibre, vitamins, minerals and enzymes as approximately 9 grams of barley grass is equal to 5 fruits and vegetables,

FAST TRACK VERSION

Here is a checklist for people who want to lose weight quickly.

- Follow The Food Voice Diet eating programme

- Reduce carbohydrate intake to the lowest level that works for you. 20-40 grams per day is the lowest level.

- Limit fruit consumption ensuring that you take the barley grass supplement to supplement any lost nutrients.

- Limit nuts to 4 per day

- Snack on barley grass twice per day

- Take cod liver oil supplement, do not exceed recommended dose

- Drink 10 glasses of water per day

- Consume enough protein do not eat under the recommended amount. The daily amount is approximately between 50-90 grams per day divided between three meals

- Use coconut oil as the main source of fat for all meals

- Start the day with bulletproof coconut tea or coffee to promote energy levels

- Do not cut down the recommended amount of coconut oil, which boosts metabolism and provides energy. This minimum daily allowance is approximately 6 teaspoons per day to include bulletproof drink and amount to cook with.

- Exercise or brisk walk three times per week for 10-20 minutes at least.

- Cut down on excess coffee, tea and alcohol

- Eat non-starchy vegetables (see the 5 carb per serving list).

- Adequate sleep

- Deal with stress more efficiently

- Do not take the one day off from low carb allowance

WHY DRINK PLENTY OF WATER

The body needs adequate water in order to burn fat as the process of burning calories only works efficiently if you are hydrated. The liver and kidneys aid fat burning and need to work efficiently. This is the reason many diets inform us we need to drink water, but they often forget to tell us why this is so important. Water also helps to maintain muscle tone, which is important in our quest for leanness and looking good. The Food Voice Diet advises that at least 10 glasses of pure water be consumed every day. If you exercise or live in a hot climate, you will need to drink more. Alcohol can cause dehydration which can affect your fat burning mechanism. Although water is not a food, it can be considered as a nutrient and is essential for optimal health. Water is required for digestion, circulation, transporting nutrients, organ protection, moisturising air in the lungs, removal of toxins, helping to keep good energy supply, regulating body temperature, muscle fuel, keeping the immune system healthy, helping to produce saliva, keeping our joints hydrated, hydrating the skin and it transports oxygen around the body, helping to reduce fatigue, keep your brain focused, reduce stress, helps fluid retention and kidney function.

The brain 90% water

Blood 83% water

Bone 22% water

Muscle 75% water

SIGNS OF DEHYDRATION

- Fatigue
- Constipation
- Lack of concentration
- Bad breath
- Muscle cramps
- Irregular blood pressure
- Kidney problems
- Dry skin
- Thirst
- Hunger
- Headache
- Affects physical performance negatively
- Feeling unwell generally or bad mood

FOODS TO AVOID

High fructose corn syrup HFCS.
This sugar product was manufactured after the Second World War as a cheaper substitute for cane sugar. It is sweeter than sugar and added to many processed sweet products, breakfast cereals and savoury foods, sauces and pickles. It is the main sugar ingredient in soda drinks such as colas. It helps to brown food enhancing its appearance. It is utilized in frozen food as a preservative and to keep the price of products as low as possible. The addition of large amount of HFCS make products more addictive as extra sugar is expected once the taste buds get used to sweet tastes. Although HFCS is a sugar substitute it is not metabolised in the body in the same way as other types of sugar as it can only be processed by

the liver. This product can cause a fatty liver and damage similar to that of alcohol abuse, as the body views it as a toxin. HFCS is made up of fructose and glucose and used in many products in high amounts providing excess glucose energy for the body to use causing fat storage. High levels of fructose put a strain on the liver, as this is a substance the liver normally metabolises in small amounts. Excess fructose is turned into fat by the liver, increasing the risk of blood triglycerides, fat storage, metabolic syndrome and gout. Experts are now linking this product to brain deterioration. You can be overeating HFCS by consuming the following; sugary breakfast cereals, sweet fruit juice drinks, sodas, sports drinks, power bars, fruit and flavoured yogurts, salad dressings, nutrition bars, crackers, biscuits, ice cream as well as many fat free and low fat products, milk chocolate and confectionery, packet stuffing, muffins, ketchup and similar sauces, cough syrups, jars of cooking sauces, pizzas, soups, canned fruits and processed ready meals

Fructose content of food

1. Regular soda 23 grams
2. Apple 10 grams
3. Blackberries 1 portion 4 grams
4. Dried fruit 1 portion 20 grams
5. I mango 15 grams
6. I kiwi 3 grams
7. Table sugar 50% fructose
8. Agave syrup is 90% fructose

- **Sugar and simple carbohydrates.**
  Empty calories with little nutritional content. The

success of The Food Voice Diet is based on reducing your carbohydrate intake and type. Eating excess carbohydrates are transformed into fat storage by your body. More insulin = more fat. Focus on complex carbohydrates with fibre, vitamins and minerals.

- **Fruit juices, sodas and soft drinks.**
  These drinks contain large amounts of sugar causing insulin spikes.

- **Trans fats**
  are liquid fats heated to a very high temperature. During the cooling process, hydrogen is added to turn liquid into solid fats. These fats are added to many processed food products partly because they are cheap, but also because they add shelf life to the product. Trans fat is so hard to digest, break down and metabolize because the product is synthetic. This is where clogged up arteries come into the picture as trans fat transports LDL cholesterol to the arteries. Trans fats and partially hydrogenated vegetable oils are found in products such as margarine, pizzas, cakes, cereals, ready meals and confectionery products. Restaurants serving deep fat fried food use trans fats as the fat keeps longer and is less expensive to buy. Maximising profit is the goal as opposed to concerns over the consumer's health. We need to be concerned and make a decision to substantially reduce or eliminate eating these products. In November 2013 the US Food and Drug Administration (FDA) declared the organisation is reviewing the use of partially hydrogenated vegetable oils as a safe ingredient for food manufacturing under the band called (GRAS) generally

recognized as safe.

- **Table salt**
is refined salt containing additives. The recommended salt intake is innocently abused when eating a large amount of processed foods as the salt is very well disguised with the sugar, flavourings, chemicals and other additives. Excess table salt can cause health issues such as high blood pressure, stroke and weight gain. Salt is added for flavour and for its preservative value. The more food is processed the more salt is generally added. Salt is added to obvious food such as ready meals and snacks like crisps, but surprisingly to sweet foods like biscuits, breakfast cereals, cola and fruit drinks. Sodium is good for us in moderation, but by eating processed foods we are over consuming unknowingly. Up to 1 tsp of unrefined salt per day is good guideline.

- **Processed food.**
Some processed foods such as milk, frozen fruit and vegetables can be a useful addition to our diet. Therefore, foods that have been minimally processed would be the best options to choose. Most tinned food can be avoided apart from tomatoes, coconut milk, tuna, and salmon (fresh is best). Beans and vegetables can be used if washed really well, but fresh or frozen vegetables are a better choice.

- **Fast food junk meals.**
These foods are always loaded with sugar, salt and the wrong type of fats and should be avoided. The worst type is the deep fat fried foods. If you do have to eat in fast

food places occasionally, skip on the soda, the fries and the extra cheese type meals. This will reduce your fat, salt and sugar overload.

- **Confectionery and sweets.**
These products contain huge amounts of sugar and often the high fructose corn syrup which is a health risk if eaten in large quantities. The problem is, if we buy these items and have them at home, we will eat them. It is easy to form a habit and become addicted to these products. Use other healthy foods as treats instead. Cupboard love is not real love, you are not being kind to yourself or your family by offering these items to them in excess.

- **Low calorie and low fat food.**
These foods are not suitable for The Food Voice Diet because they are not savoured and totally enjoyed, plus when fat is removed from a product, more sugar is added in an attempt to make the product taste better. It is possible to feel full after eating this food from the physical aspect and remain hungry from a mental point of view. You are left unsatisfied mentally and you may be subject to cravings and strong urges forcing you to overeat. Foods of this type are normally very processed and expensive. Calories are not all equal, this is very hard for many dieters to get their head around as calorie counting has been around a long time as a tool for losing weight. For example, if you consumed 1000 calories per day of carbohydrates compared to 1000 calories of protein and fat. The diet causing an insulin spike would result in the highest weight gain. Full fat milk is more beneficial as the calcium in milk is absorbed more

efficiently with vitamin D, which is contained in the fat of milk. Therefore low-fat milk contains less natural vitamin D and higher levels of lactose (milk sugar). Full fat milk slows down sugar absorption supporting blood sugar and insulin control. Food and drinks fortified with vitamins contain the synthetic type preventing proper absorption and effectiveness.

- **Ready made meals.**
These foods often contain high amounts of hidden sugar, unhealthy fat, excess salt, preservatives, synthetic flavours and chemicals that we would not normally have in home cooked food. The liver can struggle to process this food if eaten on a regular basis, which can affect your ability to burn fat and maximise your health. These meals, should only be consumed on an occasional basis.

- **Alcohol**
is hard to metabolize by the liver and can cause fatty liver. Alcohol can be sent to our cells directly, the brain processes some alcohol, which causes the buzz and intoxication. If your liver is not working effectively, it will affect your health and struggle to process the food you eat. This can contribute to weight gain. In moderation, alcohol is relaxing and an aid to socializing. However, it can cause insulin spikes as it is often served with additional sugar laden mixers. If alcohol is consumed in excess, not only are you consuming many more calories without nutrients, but alcohol can create feelings of hunger and craving for high fat, high carbohydrate and junk food. To avoid insulin spikes from the sugar in alcohol, consume it alongside a meal containing protein,

fat and fibre. Alcohol should be counted as part of your carbohydrate allowance. Hangovers are well known to trigger a desire for carbohydrates, sugar and junk food as we are making food decisions in an 'out of balance' state. Soda drink mixers are not recommended as they contain high fructose corn syrup and many additives. (See carb list for alcohol and mixers at the back of the book)

- **Genetically modified soy**
  products (GMO) are frequently associated with allergies and digestive reactions. Organic soy products can be tolerated more easily. The pesticides used for GMO are used at substantially higher levels in comparison to non GMO crops

- **Sugar substitutes and sweeteners.**
  Diet soda drinks or any food or drink sweetened artificially without the calories, trains us to want sugar. They can also contain toxic chemicals that can affect our health.

WHY EXERCISE HELPS

The Food Voice Diet motivates you to feel energised and more in the mood for movement without having to drag yourself to the gym. Lack of energy can really set us back at the thought of having to engage in activities. Feeling lethargic, finding excuses and experiencing fatigue even after sleep are all signs your diet needs changing. Relying on caffeine drinks to get through your day can really takes its toll after a few weeks by sapping your energy even more. As

166

we age, we experience the decline in digestive and metabolic enzymes, which can affect our energy levels including the type of food we eat. The Food Voice Diet includes a list of foods and supplements to help you get your energy levels up and running. On a mental level the diet helps you to feel better by getting rid of foods that stress the body out resulting in cravings and mental imbalance. You will soon feel like exercising once you change your diet, it is fine to wait until you feel more energy flowing again before you exercise when movement won't feel like such an effort. Using coconut oil as your main source of fat for one-month boosts energy levels as this oil is not digested like other fats giving you energy instead of using your energy to process it. Any food you eat which strains or overloads your system saps your energy especially, excess sugar and toxins. You can acquire your energy back giving you a new lease of life, instead of wasting it processing the wrong foods. Moderate exercise is recommended.

- Muscle uses up more energy and improves your metabolic rate. Makes us looked toned and more attractive.

- Muscle weighs more than fat. If you start to build up muscle during weight loss it can appear on the scales as a weight increase however you have lost inches.

- Helps control weight. Do not rely on exercise alone to lose weight. Avoid exercising just to burn calories so that you can eat more later. Do not use exercise as a permission slip to eat more, as you may not have burned as many calories as you think. It takes a huge amount of physical activity to burn one slice of bread. Your weight loss is best orchestrated by The Food Voice Diet style of eating.

- Improves flexibility and posture, builds bones

- Helps reduce insulin levels, boosts brain power

- Reduces toxin release, expands lung capacity.

- Stress reduction if you do not over exercise.

- Good for the heart and circulation, helps prevent diseases.

- Releases good feeling chemicals called endorphins. Improves quality of life

- Make sure you eat enough food for your energy requirements as trying to reduce your food intake can lower your metabolism, reducing activity making you feel lethargic and lazy.

- Makes us feel better mentally and physically

- Check with a doctor before exercising especially if obese to avoid injury and joint problems. It helps to concentrate on moving more and sitting less each day. Making small improvements no matter how small helps you get in the right mindset and make progress. It is best to set yourself achievable small goals to avoid letting yourself down with unrealistic targets.

DIFFICULT SITUATIONS HOW TO COPE

Being prepared for the difficult times is of huge importance. I am not suggesting you prepare for failure, but I am saying that life happens and we need to be prepared for days when we may, for whatever reason, eat the wrong food. Going off track should not be viewed as a huge negative and give you a reason to punish yourself by having an all out binge or giving up completely. When we go off track without planning, the track will be longer and make the return to balance all the more difficult. Realistically it could be said that there will be at least three occasions you know of, where you will plan to go off track, i.e. Christmas, your birthday and a holiday. There may be at least three other off days where stress gets the better of you or a life event may cause you to derail temporarily. The points to consider are:

1. Being prepared is a method of practising damage limitation as opposed to denying this will ever happen to you and are caught off guard.
2. The degree to which you over consume the wrong foods will be reduced.
3. Being aware of your decision keeps you in control and mindful

4. Making time to plan makes getting back on track much easier as you are not overwhelmed or out of control. You can then move on.
5. You can re-start your programme totally avoiding mentally beating yourself up, which causes binging and other negative food choices.

The first step is always:

"KNOW YOU ARE THE BOSS"

You are always going to be in charge of every meal and be responsible for whatever you eat. You are stronger than junk food which cannot have power over you, as long as you do not eat it on a regular basis. Note "I will just eat one" is difficult with any form of junk food as they have been designed for over indulgence and addiction.

The second step is being clear what occasional means.

OCCASIONAL FOODS

Junk food can be occasional foods, but never say they are an occasional treat. You have new treats now. It would be hard to say that for the rest of your life you will never ever eat junk food. You can even enjoy occasional junk food experiences, but know that if you allow them to be more than occasional you run the risk of addiction. What is an occasional food? Well, it is not connected to something you do on a regular basis. For example if you went to the cinema and consumed a hot dog, sweet popcorn and a cola, but did this once a week that is not occasional. If you went once or twice a year, it would pass. Allowing yourself junk foods only on occasions is an experience where you may well discover that you do not derive the same pleasure as you used to as you have got used to real food treats. The first crisp may taste OK, but after a few you may well feel like eating something else. If you eat excess junk food even occasionally it tends to leave you feeling off and you will have wished you had not indulged.

After a while, you may still eat it on occasions, but you will not want to go for excess as you used to.

TOO MANY OCCASIONS

If you have a busy social calendar, full of many events, you will have to divide your occasions into eating categories in order to avoid the excuse of saying you can eat all the wrong foods at special events and it is not your fault you have to attend so many. For example out of ten events choose two that you will eat off this diet, but for the other eight you will stay on track. The wrong thinking can give you wrong eating habits. You will have to make choices and work around the lifestyle you have. The idea is to choose only occasional events that allow occasional off track eating. If some events are more work orientated you may feel that they are in one category and family and personal events another. Anything too regular can easily become a habit. Do not deceive yourself about this and if you habitually eat junk food, you run the risk of becoming mentally and physically addicted to it. There are no short cuts, no lies you can tell yourself, no excuses. These are the cold facts. Do not eat junk foods on a regular basis. High carbohydrate meals on a regular basis cause fat storage and affect your body detrimentally.

TEMPTATIONS AND CRAVINGS

Allowing yourself the occasional indulgence removes this food from the forbidden "**must have**" category. The experience of wanting a particular food so badly it almost feels unbearable is a situation you need a plan for. If you attend a wedding telling yourself "I will not give in, I will not eat the cake, I will not eat the dessert, I will not, I will not, I will not." When you finally give in you would be more likely to stuff the food down and want more and more before you had the time to really taste the food. Out of control eating often takes place at a very fast speed as the food is hardly chewed before we shovel in the next mouthful. We can consume huge amounts in this state, which is always regretted. However, if you have given yourself permission you are much less likely to eat in such a frenzy as you can now naturally slow down and eat consciously. I have found that by allowing myself occasions to eat junk food really makes me think twice if I even want it. I now prefer my other treat foods, which I regularly consume. Not being deprived in the first place is such a major help physically and mentally by reducing the desire to eat food that does not benefit me.

NEGATIVE SELF TALK

This is a subject that needs addressing as it can take a good day and turn it into a bad one. Negative self-talk can occur over small events such as a bad day at work, a misunderstanding or making a mistake. If your diet is healthy thus providing you with nutrients to support you during stressful situations you will have greater access to inner strength and resilience. The Food Voice Diet contains some wonderfully calming comfort foods which will help soothe you, preventing you from going off track and ruining your progress. No matter how annoyed, frustrated or angry you are, consuming junk food and sugar will only make you feel worse later. Sugar and food binges give you a bigger problem than the one that sparked your discomfort in the first place. Your self-talk should incorporate a pledge that you will no longer internalize outside events by eating as the solution. You now refuse to wear negative emotions in the form of excess fat. Your new food voice will say to you something like "yes this was a tough old day, you certainly got the brunt of the manager's bad mood. You need a healthy comfort meal, remember how much you love that chicken with the creamy sauce and your favourite, avocado. You can tuck up in bed later with a hot milk and melting chocolate square and today will be a distant memory. You will wake up tomorrow feeling great and not even give this a second thought". Your old food voice would say " This is so out of order you must be furious. On your way home stop and buy chocolate and pick up a takeaway you are in no mood to cook, just picture yourself munching away on that massive bar of chocolate, you will feel much better." You follow the suggestion and by 10pm you feel so guilty about your binge, plus now you are mad at yourself and your boss and wake up tomorrow in a bad mood feeling fat.

BOREDOM

Thinking about food can arise out of boredom. In fact, you can talk yourself into believing you are hungry when really there is nothing else that springs to mind other than the fridge. Eating is not an antidote to having nothing else to do if you want to lose weight. Other quick fix solutions which will save your waistline are as follows: call a friend, link in with someone who would really benefit from your call, have a shower, play some music, watch a funny film. Eating when bored can become a habit especially if you eat the wrong diet and have a food voice which gives you food suggestions as opposed to one that will enhance your life. Your food voice should sound something like this "you are bored but if you go to the fridge now and start eating you will still be bored in ten minutes and feel worse. You have lost weight and are still adjusting to having free time in the evening when you used to eat. I tell you what would be fun, how about making a list of what you are going to buy when you reach your weight loss goal." You follow the suggestions and start to feel so motivated that the thought of going to the fridge seems absurd.

ALCOHOL

Is made of sugar and can cause excess calories to be consumed. Not only can this be a problem in terms of weight gain, but also alcohol can stimulate the appetite for carbohydrate foods during consumption and also during the hangover process. It is wise to cut back on alcohol in order to lose weight and to maintain your ideal weight. Choose drinks that do not include mixers like cola and lemonade, which increase extra sugar and toxins. Alcohol also rids the body of certain minerals and vitamins during its metabolism, which can affect your health alongside damage to the liver. In moderation and in combination with a healthy diet alcohol can be relaxing and play a part in socialising.

SELF SABOTAGE

There appears to be another general trend for people to associate the over consumption of junk foods as something to be proud of and a topic to boast about. Over indulging in the wrong type of behaviours can be attention seeking even if it is the wrong attention. People will generally laugh with you when you tell them you ate two pizzas, a packet of biscuits and two chocolate bars washed down by a large cola in one evening because you were having a bad day. Eating can be a form of social acceptance incorporating the need to behave in a certain way. People often try to sabotage your healthy eating plan, as they want company to consume the foods you are trying to avoid. Sometimes people can get quite annoyed when you say 'no' to the foods that they actually want you to eat. Misery loves company right? How many times have you heard the following:

- "Oh come on just try the cake you can start your diet tomorrow"
- "Don't be boring ...you look fine as you are"
- "I have made this especially for you"
- "Just finish off this I don't want it to go to waste"
- "Have a day off, start again tomorrow"

Healthy eaters can be ridiculed and seen as un-cool or geeks. Young children and teens are particularly vulnerable to this type of social acceptance. The same people who shared your joke will not be as interested when you tell them that you spent the next day hating yourself and were upset and disgusted about your binge and now feel depressed. No one wants to hear the real story of your eating issues or how miserable being overweight feels. Realize that although your friend may laugh at your over indulgence it really is not a joke to you. If you feel uncomfortable informing people you have changed your diet...don't. They may not even notice that you no longer have any more binge stories to tell them but what they really notice is how good you are looking instead.

FEAR OF LETTING GO OF CERTAIN FOODS

If you are feeling anxious and finding it hard to say goodbye to certain habits, patterns or a particular food then it would be best to build this into your programme until you feel you can let go. The main rule to remember is not to eat carbohydrate without protein, to avoid sugar spikes and fat storage.

DISAPPOINTMENT YOU NO LONGER ENJOY CERTAIN FOODS

When the foods you really used to love to eat no longer have the same effect, you may feel a sense of loss. Now, when you attempt to indulge in your once favourite chocolate bar or cake it feels disappointing. It is quite normal to have these feelings as it is part of the process of change. Focus more on your new treats and you will be able to move on as going back is not an option you choose.

IS IT NORMAL TO USE FOOD AS SOMETHING TO LOOK FORWARD TO?

The Food Voice Diet promotes looking forward to eating the healthy food, which supports you. Each meal and drink should be thoroughly enjoyed and savoured. Allowing yourself this pleasure satisfies not just your appetite but your brain. Eating this way blunts any further desire to eat, thoughts of extra food you fancy disappear from your universe. Your food voice goes quiet. When you are full, but are still on the look out for food this is your brain talking to you. To ensure this voice switches off after you eat make sure the food you eat also feeds your brain which then leaves you in peace and satisfied.

We will never be able to live just eating for survival or to simply satisfy hunger, we have evolved way beyond these basic requirements. Choosing a food reward is healthy under the right conditions. We are asking too much of ourselves if we try to deny ourselves pleasure from eating. You could fill yourself up on low fat food you do not really enjoy until you could burst, but your brain will tell you something is missing, you may well hear your cupboards talking to you. Will power does not work, as eventually you will have to seek out that treat you have been denying yourself even if you have to drive to the nearest shop you will. We have to eat so why not make the food tasty and something we look forward to as it really does make your day more enjoyable. Be wise and kind to yourself by planning your treats and rewards, but choose the ones that are not addictive. We are programmed to eat for pleasure, relish the food you eat safe in the knowledge that by following this diet you will not experience the post food guilt trip once the last mouthful finishes.

WHAT TO DO IF YOU GO OFF TRACK

Going off track on the odd occasion is not going to ruin your waistline forever nor does it mean you have failed and therefore trigger you into going even more off track. Punishing yourself by overeating or coping by overeating can occur from time to time, but do not think you are destined to go back to your old ways. It means what you decide it means, as you are the boss here. You do not have to veer off track for days and days, as you know it will not help you. Accept the detour and get back on track the next day. You can quickly grasp control by limiting your carbohydrates the next day to less than you normally consume in order to catch back up. Make sure you do not forget to eat your treat foods to keep feeling good especially when life is tough. Your food voice may say to you "Let's make a plan for tomorrow and move on from today, it is good you do not feel good about the detour which shows you how far you have come. You have all the correct foods in the fridge to wake up to and start over. Have a great breakfast with your bullet proof coffee, take lunch to work and the evening meal can go in the slow cooker. End of detour!"

WEIGHT LOSS PLATEAU

We normally lose weight easily at the beginning of a new diet before we reach a plateau where we stop losing weight as fast or not at all. This is perfectly normal, as our body needs time to adjust to the new weight after the initial loss. Do not give up or get disappointed that all is lost. It is important to keep going and do not try to take short-cuts by cutting out healthy fats or eating less protein than your body needs or giving up carbohydrate to try to force your body to respond. Short cuts work against your goal and only lead to lowered metabolism, fatigue and lack of good mental health. Your body will adjust at the right time, you need to be patient and allow the process to work. Check the following to make sure you are on track.

1. Are you drinking enough water?
2. Have you started to drink more caffeine than normal?
3. Are you under more stress than previous weeks?
4. Have you made any dietary changes or relaxed The Food Voice Diet recommendations?
5. Are you snacking more?
6. Have you missed meals or not eating enough or have taken short-cuts?

WEANING YOURSELF OFF CERTAIN FOODS

The Food Voice Diet is an eating plan you can grow into if you are currently unable to make a full commitment to the diet for your own personal reasons.
"A journey of a thousand miles begins with a single step" Lao Tzu

The first step is make the initial adjustments which are:

• Never eat carbohydrates without protein and fat to slow down the insulin response.

- More insulin = more fat, keeps the carbs down!
- You will eat less of any problem foods if you consume them after dinner as opposed to when you are hungry.
- Add at least one extra healthy food per day.
- Set a limit to your adjustment period and make sure you are making progress by cutting down the problem foods each week or each day.
- Drink the water allowance
- Take the cod liver oil and barley grass
- Start reading through the steps 1-14 and complete as much of the list as possible.
- Try a "one day on" The Food Voice Diet and "one day off" and then "two days on" and "one day off,"
- Gradually increase the number of days on until you are fully on board.

THE FOOD VOICE DIET AFFIRMATIONS

1   "It is so clear now that my second helpings were my downfall. I now release the old conditioning of my childhood. I know that eating that much food does not work for me, it is detrimental to my health and happiness. I am no longer a child and I now choose to make adult decisions to help myself lose weight."

2   "I will not be influenced by advertising and eat what the manufactures of junk foods want me to eat. I choose what I know is right and healthy for me."

3   "I am not afraid to stand up for myself and will no longer want to please other people by eating the wrong foods when offered to me."

4   "I am happy to know that foods which caused insulin spikes were to blame for my weight gain. I have moved on from overeating pasta and bread, I am in control of my appetite in a way I have never experienced before"

5   "I am finding other ways to deal with my negative emotions such as stress, and off days, using food only makes things much worse."

6   "I agree that I can find other things to fill up the time I spent when junk food was my hobby. This hobby was bad news and made me very unhappy and overweight."

7   "I release all blame to the food I was given as a child and the habits I have carried on as an adult. The people who love me were only doing what they thought was right at the time. I can change this now as the power is in the present not the past."

8   "I am making my list of new food treats, junk food is not a treat as it has not done me any favours. I can change that now. I will not ignore the fact that I am designed for rewards and I will no longer go on deprivation diets or eat in ways that do not support my happiness and mental balance."

9   "I allow myself to lose the excess weight and keep it off. I am giving instructions to my fat cells to release the

excess weight which does not belong to me. This is a real final goodbye, not I will see you later type of intention. I am not losing the weight to find it again as this really is the grand send off. This weight has no place in my life, it was acquired through the wrong thoughts and incorrect information. I now know better, with the new knowledge I have acquired, I can really make The Food Voice Diet work."

10   "I am willing to learn the new habits, as I really want to let go of the past and my old way of eating. I want to replace my junk food eating for something that will make me happy in the short and long term. I no longer want to suffer with lack of confidence about my shape."

11   "I am changing my unhealthy diet for this new plan that will work for me. I am ready, there is nothing holding me back, I am cutting out junk food in order to fit into my old clothes again. I plan to go out more and get my life back."

12   "I am not allowing my brain to become addicted to junk foods which it will if I do not make the right choices. I no longer deny this fact and see this type of food as harmless."

STEPS TO STARTING THE DIET

We have now arrived at the starting line to help you find your new food voice for weight loss.

There is some minor list writing involved, but it will come in so handy on the days when you cannot think what to eat or you are stuck in a rut. Making your list will really help you stay on track and remind you what you love to eat.

STEP 1

Now is the time, if you have not already done so, to write down the main problem areas you want to work on from the following list. What really is your downfall when it comes to losing weight?

- My portions are too large
- I eat all the food on my plate, hungry or not
- I eat to relax or deal with emotions
- I eat excessive amounts of junk food
- I crave certain foods - write them down
- I am constantly hungry
- I think too much about food
- I eat too much sugar
- I skip meals and then overeat
- I eat out of boredom

STEP 2

What time of day is the most difficult for you in terms of overeating and choosing the wrong food?
Write down the area you would like to work on and the time of day you need support by having a new food treat you really like, which is not junk food. The worst time of day for most people is in the evening. This will help you in the initial stage of the diet when you need more support. This is a learning curve and progress will be made but not overnight. Allow yourself the time to change.

What occasions and triggers normally make you lose control? Prepare in advance for when you are prone to need a treat to keep you going or as a pick me up. Eating often has nothing to do with being hungry, be prepared for these situations in advance. Once you have a list of new treat foods and you get used to eating them you will not feel old craving and urges so strongly. Our lives can be quite mundane at times and we need to have food and snacks to look forward to, which do not compromise our weight and happiness. Out of habit, we reach for the old-fashioned sugar or junk food snack simply because we have never thought of any other choices. We do not have to eat junk food to have a treat. Once you get used to eating treats that are not junk food, the other food has less appeal.

Plan your treat into the part of your day when you are normally prone to overeating such as:

- Watching TV
- Getting the children's meal and homework sorted out
- Leaving work and having to commute home
- Feeling tired in the afternoon
- Eating whilst preparing the family meal

By planning your treats for the day, you will already be feeling better and you may even be able to delay your treat until you can sit down and really enjoy a well-earned break. Often the mere fact that you can plan and have treats helps you feel more controlled and peaceful about food in general. Your new food voice will help you negotiate the correct food choice for example "I normally have my bar of chocolate watching my favourite programme this is ideal for tonight" changes to "For my meal tonight I am going to cook my absolute favourite meal and then go for the dark chocolate as my dessert. It ticks all the right boxes so I do not have to worry I am going to want to binge."

STEP 3

* Write down your current weight,
* Decide on how much weight you would like to lose.
* If you do not know your weight, write down how you would like to look or what size clothes you would like to wear.

STEP 4

Have a good clear out of your food cupboards and refrigerator.

STEP 5

Write out your list of the foods you love to eat which do not include junk food. Try to make this list as long as possible. It is very easy to hit a blank when we think of what to have for dinner. This list should be making your mouth water whilst you are writing.

STEP 6

Write a list of sauces, flavours and seasoning you really like to use when cooking. What would make a piece of cooked chicken or salmon taste extra special to you? What makes your mouth water? This is a good list to refer to when you are in a rush and want to enjoy a healthy meal, but feel you have had a treat too.

STEP 7

Make a list of some short cuts that you can take when you do not have time to cook or cannot face it. This will help to stop you going off track.

STEP 8

Make a list of vegetables that you like and how you like them cooked. Include a variety of salads but only if you really enjoy it.

STEP 9

Snacks are important especially in the beginning of the diet when you may still be experiencing cravings and adjusting to the diet. Nuts are ideal. If the nuts are salted you can rub the majority of salt off with a paper towel. Remember do not eat any carbohydrate on its own for a snack always include some protein. Choose snacks that you really enjoy, but not junk food. The barley grass drink is brilliant for taking the edge of hunger, whilst providing you with protein, vitamins, minerals and enzymes. It is a brilliant choice for a weight loss snack.

STEP 10

Book your medical check up.

STEP 11

Choose a form of exercise even if is only walking if you are not currently engaged in an activity. Decide to move more and sit less.

STEP 12

Shopping list to start The Food Voice Diet

Organic coconut oil. Do not buy hydrogenated coconut oil. Add grass fed butter and any other recommended oils.

- Order cod liver oil and barley grass powder
- Check list of favourite food and buy enough meat or fish for the following week
- Stock up the freezer with organic fruit and vegetables
- Plan breakfast menu for the next week and put items on the list.
- If lunching at work make a plan for the next week, where to eat or what food to take with you.
- Plan a couple of slow cooker meals for the busiest days of the week
- Buy containers to carry snacks in including barley grass, nuts and coconut oil
- Plan to cook a few meals for the freezer whenever possible
- Make soup with bones from meat or fish
- Buy enough mineral water for the following week

STEP 13

Download the food list. Charts from the website.
www.thefoodvoicediet.com
The Food Voice Diet recipe book will be published in 2014.

STEP 14

Measure waist circumference if you wish to chart your progress
(see key 5)

	Ideal	Average	Too high
Women	Under 31.5 inches (80 cm)	1.5 – 35 inches (80 – 88 cm)	Over 35 inches (88 cm)
Men	Under 37 inches (94 cm)	37 – 40 inches (94 - 102 cm)	Over 40 inches (102 cm)

"NEVER, NEVER, NEVER GIVE UP"
Winston Churchill

The Food Voice Diet Recommended Food List			
Food Description	Serving	Approx Carbs grams	Approx Protein grams
Milk,cream and dairy			
Coconut milk	100g	2.6	1.3
Full Fat Plain Yogurt	100g	5	3
Greek Yogurt	100g	3.65	9
Milk (Whole)	100g	4.8	3.3
Sour Cream	100g	4.27	3.6
Whipping Cream	100g	2.8	2.05
Raw milk	1 cup	12	8
Eggs	1	Trace	12.5
Cheese			
Cheddar	100g	1.3	24.9
Camembert	100g	0.5	19.5
Edam	100g	1.4	24.9
Feta	100g	4.1	14.21
Gruyère	100g	0.4	29.81
Monterey	100g	0.68	24.48
Mozzarella	100g	3.1	27.5
Parmesan	100g	4.06	38.46
Ricotta	100g	5.0	11.39
Swiss	100g	5.38	26.93

Goats	100g	1.87	23.52
Cottage cheese	100g	2.86	12.40
Grains and Pasta			
Bagel plain	100g	50.5	10.02
Coconut flour	100g	65	19
Cous cous	100g	73.1	15.1
Gluten free bread	100g	56	11.8
Multi Grain Bread	100g	43.3	13.5
Oatmeal	100g	66.7	16.89
Pancake	100g	28.3	6.4
Pasta	100g	33	5.1
Quinoa	100g	68.9	13.1
Rice	100g	28.5	2.38
Rye Bread	100g	48.3	8.5
Spaghetti - whole wheat	100g	26.5	5.3
Pita Bread whole-wheat	100g	55	9.8
White Bread	100g	50	0
Tortilla	100g	46.6	5.7

The Food Voice Diet Recommended Food List			
Food Description	Serving	Approx Carbs grams	Approx Protein grams
Grains and Pasta			
Egg Noodles	100g	25.16	4.54
1 Slice bread		15	
Wholemeal bread	100g	47	9.13
Pita bread	100g	50.1	9.6
Bulgur Wheat	100g	18.5	3.06
Yorkshire Pudding	100g	38	9
Meat, Poultry and Fish			
Beef	100g	0	21.2
Veal	100g	0	26
Chicken	100g	0	18.5
Lamb	100g	0	24.2
Pork	100g	0.88	19.4
Bacon	100g	0	15.9
Beef Salami	100g	0	15.9
Duck	100g	0	11.5
Ham/Gammon	100g	0	26.8
Sausages (Beef)	100g	3.99	11.04
Sausages (Pork)	100g	0	15.09

Pheasant	100g	0	32.26
Calves Liver	100g	3.9	19.9
Seafood			
Anchovies	100g		20
Clams	100g	2.57	12.77
Fish Roe	100g	1.5	22.3
Lobster	100g	3.12	26.41
Oysters	100g	9.9	18.9
Prawn	100g	0.3	17.09
Scallops	100g	2.36	16.8
Shrimp	100g	0.9	13.6
Mackerel	100g	0	19.31
Cod	100g	0	17.81
Tuna	100g	0	23.38
Sardines	100g	0	24.58
Crab	100g	0	20.3
Soups - Homemade			
Beef stock soup	100g	1.2	2
Chicken soup	100g	3.88	1.68
Beef marrow bone	100g	0	29.87
Pork marrow bone	100g	0	28.6
Miso soup	100g	3.24	2.51

The Food Voice Diet Recommended Food List			
Food Description	Serving	Approx Carbs grams	Approx Protein grams
Vegetables			
Artichoke	100g	10.87	3.37
Asparagus	100g	3.88	2.2
Aubergine	100g	6	1
Bean Sprouts	100g	6	3.2
Broccoli	100g	3.2	4.2
Brussel Sprouts	100g	8.95	3.38
Cabbage	100g	9.6	0.9
Carrot	100g	7.9	0.6
Cauliflower	100g	5.3	1.9
Celery	100g	3	1.98
Chillies	100g	9.14	1.94
Corn	100g	19.02	3.22
Courgette	100g	3.35	1.21
Cucumber	100g	3.63	0.65
Endive	100g	3.4	1.3
Garlic	100g	33.06	6.36
Leek	100g	14	1.5
Lettuce	100g	2.9	1.4
Lettuce (Romaine)	100g	3.3	1.2

Mushroom	100g	3.9	2.1
Okra	100g	7.5	1.9
Onion	100g	9.3	1.1
Peas	100g	7.6	2.8
Peppers	100g	4.6	0.9
Potato	100g	17.2	2.1
Pumpkin	100g	8.09	1.1
Radish	100g	3.4	0.68
Runner Beans	100g	7.13	1.82
Sauerkraut	100g	4.28	0.92
Spinach	100g	3.3	1.1
Squash	100g	3.9	1
Tomato	100g	3.0	0
Turnips	100g	6.4	0.9
Yam	100g	27.9	1.5
Watercress	100g	1.29	2.3

The Food Voice Diet Recommended Food List			
Food Description	Serving	Approx Carbs grams	Approx Protein grams
Beans			
Black Beans	100g	23.71	8.86
Butter beans	100g	20.17	6.84
Chick peas	100g	.27	9
Lentils	100g	57	28
Red Kidney	100g	61	22.5
Peanuts	2 tbsp	3.4	4.7
Fruit			
Apple	100g	14	0.26
Apricots	100g	11	1.4
Avocado	100g	9	1.09
Banana	100g	23	1.2
Blueberries	100g	14	1
Cantaloupe melon	100g	8	0.84
Cherries	100g	9	0.77
Figs	100g	19	0.75
Grapes Red/ Green	100g	18.1	0.72
Honeydew Melon	100g	9	0.54
Lemon	100g	10.7	1.2
Orange	100g	15.5	1.3

Tomato	100g	4.	1
Kiwi fruit	100g	15	1.14
Mango	100g	17	0.51
Olives	100g	3.84	1.03
Orange	100g	8.5	1.1
Peach	100g	19.7	0.54
Pear	100g	15	0.38
Pineapple	100g	13	0.54
Plum	100g	11.42	0.7
Raspberries	100g	12	1.2
Strawberries	100g	23.53	0.56
Tangerine	100g	9.5	0.62
Water Melon	100g	7.5	0.4
Nuts and Seeds			
Almonds	100g	6.9	21.1
Brazil Nuts	100g	12	14.82
Coconut – desiccated	100g	23.7	6.9
Hazelnuts	100g	17	14.95
Macadamia	100g	14	7.91
Pecan	100g	13.5	9.5

The Food Voice Diet Recommended Food List			
Food Description	Serving	Approx Carbs grams	Approx Protein grams
Pine Nuts	100g	13.08	13.69
Pistachio Nuts	100g	28	21.3
Pumpkin Seeds	2 tbsp	3.1	4.2
Walnuts	100g	10	24.06
Oils/Dressings			
Mayonnaise	1 tsp	0.1	0.1
Salsa	100g	6.24	1.7
Vinegar	100g	0.04	0
Sauces			
Gravy	1 cup	11.21	8.74
Hollandaise	1 tbsp	0.29	0.77
Marmite	½ tsp	0	2
Pesto sauce	1 tbsp	0.76	2.71
Soy	1 tbsp	1.22	1
Worcestershire	1 tbsp	3.31	0
Miscellaneous			
Dark chocolate	1 oz	16	
Hummus	2 tbsp	15	
Nut Butter	2 tsp		8
Cocoa	2 tsp	10	

Soft Drinks (not recommended)			
Type	Measure	Carbs	Protein
Apple juice	100ml	11.5	0
Cola	100ml	10g	0
Cranberry juice	100ml	13.52g	0.2
Ginger Ale	100ml	8.77	0
Tonic Water	100ml	8.8	0
Orange Juice	100ml	10	1

Alcohol (not recommended)			
Type	Measure	Carb	Protein
Red wine	100ml	2.5	0.1
White wine (dry)	100ml	0.6	0.1
Rose wine	100ml	1.4	0.3
Champagne	100ml	2.27	0.7
Brandy	100ml	Trace	0
Gin	100ml	0	0
Whisky	100ml	0	0
Rum	100ml	trace	0
Vodka	100ml	trace	0
Southern Comfort	100ml	5.1	0
Port	100ml	12	0.1
Beer	Half litre	12g	0.5
Cider	Half litre	13g	0.6
Lager	Half litre	3.1	0

HIGH CARBOHYDRATE FOODS NOT RECOMMENDED		
Food Description	Serving	Approx Carbs grams
Puffed Wheat	100g	90.9
Cornflakes	100g	87.11
Bran flakes	100g	80.4
Crisps	100g	49.74
Chocolate milk	100g	10.34
Burger, chips and cola	300g	77
Milk Chocolate	43g	26
Low fat yogurt	100g	7.04
Chocolate cookie	100g	59.1
Ready meal i.e. lasagne	297g	44.0
Whole wheat biscuit	100g	46.22
Tinned soup (creamed)	100g	15
Plain or butter milk biscuit	100g	44.6
Meat pie	425g	32
Ginger bread cake	100g	49.2
Tinned peaches in syrup	1 serving	47g
Rice pudding	100g	26.62
Vanilla ice-cream	100g	23.6
Chocolate ice-cream	100g	28.2
Treacle sponge pudding	100g	50.5
French fries	100g	35.66

Disclaimer

This publication was written to provide helpful information and every effort has been made to ensure accuracy. The author has no intention to diagnose, treat or cure health problems and recommends that medical advice be sought for all health issues. Medical advice is also recommended prior to starting this diet. The Food Voice Diet represents the personal views, based on the author's experience and extensive research. The author advises that you read all the information provided on the manufacturers product labels and all food items recommended in this book, as the author is not responsible for your use of any of these products. The author disclaims all liability arising directly or indirectly from use or application of any information contained in this book.